Not My Son, Lord!

Other books by Glen Robinson

52 Things to Do on the Sabbath

If Tomorrow Comes

Not My Son, Lord!

A father's prayer for change in his son's life becomes a desperate cry to save it.

A True Story

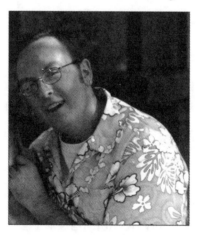

GLEN ROBINSON

Pacific Press® Publishing Association
Nampa, Idaho
Oshawa, Ontario, Canada
www.pacificpress.com

Designed by Dennis Ferree
Photos supplied by author

Copyright © 2005 by
Pacific Press® Publishing Association
Printed in the United States of America
All rights reserved

Additional copies of this book are available by
calling toll free 1-800-765-6955 or visiting
http://www.adventistbookcenter.com.

Library of Congress Cataloging-in-Publication Data

Robinson, Glen, 1953-
Not my son, Lord: a father's prayer for change in his son's life
becomes a desperate cry to save it/Glen Robinson.
p. cm.
ISBN: 0-8163-2068-3
1. Brain damage—Patients. 2. Brain damage—Patients—
Biography. 3. Head—Wounds and injuries—Patients—
Biography. 4. Head—Wounds and injuries—Patients—
Family relationships. I. Title.

RC387.5.R626 2005
617.4'81044'092—dc22   2004060768

05 06 07 08 · 5 4 3 2 1

Dedication

This book is dedicated to prayer warriors everywhere. Your ministry and compassion are the stuff miracles are made of.

Contents

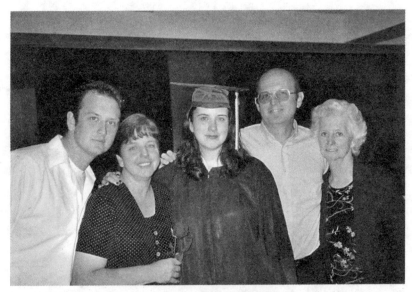

May 25, 2001, Matt, Shelly, Missy, Glen, and Nanny (before the accident)

Prologue

Caldwell, Idaho, March 12, 1997

"You two don't understand," Matt says. "You never understand!"

We are sitting on the deck outside our kitchen, talking about college. The lights of Bogus Basin Ski Resort glow on the distant hills. Matt is his usual petulant self, frustrated that he is not getting his way, determined not to take No for an answer.

"I do understand," I tell him. "You just don't want to hear what I have to say." I look up at the strong, young man who stands with fire in his eyes. It is only through the grace of God and the patience of the saints, I often think, that he has survived the academy years. He, as well as his parents. There is much good in him—and many rough edges that still need to be refined.

"Your mom and I agree that you can go to Seattle for college instead of to Walla Walla," I say. "We've talked about it, and we think you need to get out where you can sort out what you really believe. We are at least willing to try that for a while."

I remember the words of the head elder of our congregation. "I would worry about most young people moving out on their own to Seattle. But I am not worried about Matt." It is good that someone else has confidence in him.

Our decision to let Matt study at the Art Institute of

Not My Son, Lord!

Seattle instead of Walla Walla College is based partially on his struggle with reading. The Art Institute promises more emphasis on hands-on technical training, which would give Matt a greater chance for success. The other part of our decision is my own conviction that many who grow up in Adventist circles never allow their Christianity to be truly challenged. Without challenging those beliefs, it is possible to be an Adventist without knowing what it means to be a Christian.

"What about the car?" Matt asks. He stands above Shelly and me, his hands on his hips. "You just don't understand how important a nice car is to me."

I look down toward the beat-up old Ford Courier pickup I had given him this past year. Cars are simply a form of transportation to me, a hunk of metal on wheels. I don't understand his need to present himself to the world through the vehicle he drives.

"We will co-sign for a used car for you, Matthew," Shelly says from her chair beside me. "But we have to approve it. It can be something sporty, but not with heavy horsepower. And you will have to make the payments on it."

Matt nods eagerly. "I promise you won't be disappointed," he says.

I look over at Shelly. I hope not.

Key West, Florida, Christmas Eve, 2001

The warm Gulf water laps against my chest. I stand with my arms outstretched, trying to avoid stepping on the little colorful plant/animal things I see on the sandy bottom. I am standing a quarter mile from shore, and yet the water is only chest deep—and crystal clear.

Matt roars by on the Jet Ski® he and I have rented. The vacation in Florida is to celebrate my completion of classes as a doctoral student and Matt's completion of classes for his B.A. degree in communication at Southwestern Adventist University. The girls—Shelly and Missy—are spending the day in town, enjoying shopping without the two guys to slow them down.

A novel way to spend Christmas Eve, I think, as Matt draws close to me. "Your turn," he shouts and hops off the side of the big machine. I climb onto the back, gingerly. The black seat feels warm between my legs. Matt strips the life vest from his body and throws it to me to put on.

As I struggle into the vest, I am reminded that Matt's completion of school signals that he will likely be moving soon to begin his career in video production. His early idealistic dream of going to film school and becoming a film director has recently given way to a new pragmatism. Now his priority is getting a job in his field, preferably somewhere near his friends.

"A person is only as good as the friendships he has," Matt has told me time and again. People often say that we look alike and that he has many of my traits, but this is one area where we are different. I have always enjoyed friends and friendship, but I never let them keep me from pursuing my career. I suspect that Matt will soon want to move back to Idaho or on to Portland, where many of his friends from the Northwest have settled.

Is this the last vacation the four of us will have together?

Cleburne, Texas, March 4, 2002

"Well, how did it go?" I ask Matt as he strides in through the kitchen door.

He sighs. "Well, we had lots of people there. Many of them thought the loft was great." He shakes his head. "But they all pretty much said that Cleburne was too far to drive when they had to work in Fort Worth."

Not My Son, Lord!

"So, what now?" I ask. Matt looks discouraged. I know he loves living in his loft, and he even invested time and money into fixing it up when his landlord could care less how nice it looked. Everything had been fine until his roommate, Mike, had decided he couldn't afford the rent and moved out. Now Matt has twice the rent to pay, a difficult task on the wages of a restaurant server. His recent party had been an attempt to recruit a new roomie.

"Well, I'm not ready to give up yet," Matt says, as predictable as ever. "I love that place. I am sure I can find someone else who loves it as well."

"Well, just remember, you can always move back home if it gets too tough," I remind him.

Keene, Texas, April 28, 2002

Gina strides into my office at the campus radio station, throwing herself into one of the chairs. She is totally comfortable with our entire family, due to a combination of her working for me for four years and having dated Matt for almost two years.

I finish typing the public-service announcement I have on my computer and send it to print.

"How are you, Gina?" I say matter of factly, without looking up.

"Terrible," she says. I look up at her and realize that she looks terrible too.

"I wanted you to know that Matt and I broke up," she says, her face unusually sober.

"I'm sorry," I say, after a pause. *Was this predictable?* I ask myself. Their relationship had been on-again, off-again for a long time. She is a traditional Iowa girl who wants a home and Midwestern living. Matt always talks about life in the fast lane.

"The main reason was that he and I were going in different directions," she says. "The last straw was the party he threw at the loft. He was serving alcohol over there because his friends expected it. I called him on it, telling him it was wrong. And he told me 'too bad.' So I left."

I think of this and other reports of him drinking with friends. He had remained a nondrinker in Seattle for two years, while roommates drank and smoked pot around him. Now, when he is surrounded by Adventists and a loving family, he starts drinking.

"Gina, you know you will always be welcome in our house," I tell her sincerely. "But I don't blame you for wanting something more. I hope you find it."

I stare at my computer screen after Gina leaves, the words on the electronic page meaningless blips before my eyes. Finally I close my eyes in prayer, repeating a prayer I had presented before God time and again in the past few years:

God, give Matt a road-to-Damascus experience. Confront him in such a way that he cannot deny Your existence. Make him choose the path he will take for once and for all.

I slowly turn my mind back to other matters. Little did I know that the answer to my prayer would come within months—and in a way no one would expect.

CHAPTER one

The two sports cars bulleted south down I-35W, leaving Fort Worth behind them. Mike's cream-colored Mitsubishi Eclipse took turns leading and following Matt's silver turbo-charged Mazda Miata. Matt laughed joyously—and he had reasons to be happy. He was finally through with school, a bachelor's degree under his belt, and was headed out to Portland, Oregon, to look for work.

The Indian summer sun made it perfect weather to drive with the top down on his way home from work as a server at Olive Garden Italian Restaurant. Traffic was light. Matt let off on the accelerator and felt the warm wind blow through his hair. After years of being confined by parents, school, and rules, he was ready to take on the world—on his own terms. A tiny buzz tickled him inside. Was it fear of the unknown—or excitement over the limitless possibilities?

As he passed the Burleson Rest Area on his right, Matt's eye caught a light-colored car pull up on his left. Mike. Matt turned his head to face Mike's Eclipse and began to shout something. Instead, he saw Mike's eyes open wide and saw him frantically point ahead of Matt's Miata. Matt looked ahead to see his car rapidly closing in on a slow-moving diesel truck that had appeared out of nowhere into the lane in front of him.

Not My Son, Lord!

Instinctively, Matt's right foot hit the brake. The antilock braking system kept the wheels from locking up, but the Miata shuddered as it started to slow from its eighty-miles-per-hour speed. The truck, creeping along as it tried to accelerate from the rest area, loomed ahead in Matt's view. The mathematics of speed, inertia, and distance combined in an objective formula conspired against Matt and his Miata. The tiny car smashed into the back of the tractor-trailer rig at almost full speed.

My fingers flew across the keyboard. I was waiting for Matt to come home and would then take him to the airport. In the meantime, as a college professor, a radio station manager, and a doctoral student, I was taking advantage of the quiet time to get some work done.

The portable phone rang. This time, I had had the foresight to bring it to the computer instead of having to walk the twenty paces to its station in the kitchen. I answered it.

"Glen, this is Mike. Matt's been in an accident," the voice told me.

My first reaction was one of resignation. *Not again,* I thought. Matt had been in numerous fender-benders in Idaho, Washington state, and here in Texas. *His insurance rates are going to be through the roof.*

"How bad is it?"

"He's bleeding pretty bad from the face." I noticed Mike sounded panicked, and Mike was *never* excited. "He was having trouble breathing, but I held his head up, and he seems to be doing better. Paramedics are on their way."

This was sounding worse and worse.

"Where are you?" I asked.

"We were going south on I-35W, just by the Burleson Rest Area."

CHAPTER *one*

By this time, my pulse had quickened and my thinking went into crisis mode. "OK, I will be there right away," I said, and hung up.

I looked around me. *What do I need to take with me?* My mind went blank. The only thing I could think of was that if Matt was headed to the hospital, we would probably need some phone numbers of people to call. I looked for the family's black phone directory, but couldn't find it. Instead, I grabbed the bulky local phone book.

Missy was on the living room couch, watching TV.

"Matt's been in an accident over on I-35 by the rest area," I told her quickly. "Call Mom and let her know what's going on. I am headed over there now and will meet the two of you at the hospital."

"Which hospital?" she asked.

"I don't know," I stammered, then ran out the door.

Where is my cell phone? I wondered. I realized I had left it on my desk. *Do I take the time to stop and get it?* I asked myself. No, the first priority was getting to the crash site before Matt left in the ambulance. I started my Ford Ranger, threw it into reverse, and sped out of the driveway.

Mike heard a loud crunch behind him as his Eclipse sped past the eighteen-wheeler, and his heart caught in his throat. He veered over to the right past the front of the now-stopped truck, put his car in reverse, and backed up on the shoulder to where Matt's Miata lay jammed into the back of the truck.

The I-beam that served as the truck's back bumper was high enough to catch the Miata on the upper edge of the engine well. It peeled the hood and both fenders back like a can opener, folding the silver metal back all the way to the windshield. From the steering wheel back, the car was in pristine condition. From that point forward, it was a crumpled mess.

As he ran over to Matt, Mike saw the shattered windshield and saw that Matt had hit it with the knuckles of his right hand. The metal rim above the windshield was dented where Matt's forehead had struck it, even though the airbag had evidently deployed. Matt lay crumpled forward and to his right side. He was choking. Vomit dripped from his mouth. Mike reached forward and grabbed Matt's head and straightened him up. That seemed to help him breathe.

Blood poured from Matt's face, right above his eyes. Already, both eyes were beginning to swell. Mike grabbed a handkerchief from his pocket and held it against Matt's face to staunch the flow of blood.

Mike looked around and saw that traffic was beginning to back up. He saw two people on cell phones and overheard enough to know that at least one was calling 911. At that point, Mike took a minute to call me. A sedan pulled up and a large man in overalls got out and started directing traffic. Another stepped forward and introduced himself as a county deputy sheriff. He helped Mike keep Matt comfortable and started to ask questions.

After what seemed like an eternity later, but probably was only ten minutes, an ambulance arrived. Paramedics walked quickly over to the Miata and took over from the deputy and Mike, asking them to step back. Mike walked back to his Eclipse, parked on the shoulder of the interstate, and called Gina, letting her know what was happening. By that time, the paramedics had told him that Matt would be taken to Harris Methodist Hospital in Fort Worth. Mike told her to go directly there, so she would be there when Matt arrived.

CHAPTER one

"It's an accident," the teenage girl said, looking out the passenger window of the station wagon. "Looks like a bad one." Traffic was backed up for a long way.

Her mother was strangely quiet. "Honey, I have a strange feeling we should pray for whoever's in that accident. Whoever it is, they have loved ones too."

They bowed their heads and prayed.

Knowing that the accident was on the southbound side of the freeway, I chose not to get on the freeway at all. Instead I turned on the frontage road west of the freeway and sped the couple of miles to the accident site. I realized that there was no southbound traffic on the freeway. I came over a rise and then saw that cars were backed up all the way to the horizon. Ahead of me, I saw a diesel truck parked in the right lane on the interstate, a CareFlite helicopter in front of it with its rotors still turning, an ambulance, and behind that, Matt's crumpled car.

I found a place to park on the frontage road and hiked across the grass divider to the ambulance. Matt lay on a wheeled stretcher behind the ambulance. Blood made his white shirt red. Half a dozen medical personnel stood around him, working on him. *Why aren't they going to the hospital?* I wondered.

A big man with overalls and a badge stopped me before I could get to the ambulance. "That's my son!" I cried, but he pushed me back. "Let them do their work," he responded.

"Glen!" I heard behind me and was relieved to see Mike standing by his car. I joined him, and he explained how the accident had happened.

"Where's the truck driver?" I asked, raising my eyebrows.

"In the truck," Mike muttered. "The cops took a statement from him, but he never got out."

"Maybe the sheriff told him to stay put," I offered.

I walked over to the sheriff's car. The sheriff sat in the driver's seat talking to another officer. I stood for a while, trying to get their attention, but I was completely ignored. Mike walked up behind me. "The paramedics just told me that they are flying Matt out to the trauma center. If you leave now, you will get there about the time they do."

"Where is Harris Methodist?" I asked. Fort Worth is a big town.

"Off of Roseberg or Rosemont, something like that," Mike said.

"Are you the driver's father?" the overalled officer said to me, standing beside me. I turned to him and nodded. He responded by tearing a slip off of a pad and handing it to me. I stared at it blankly.

"What is it?" Mike asked.

"It's a ticket," I said numbly. "A ticket for Matt's failure to control speed."

Thirty minutes later, I entered the emergency unit lobby at Harris Methodist Hospital. "Are you Mr. Robinson?" a woman standing behind the glass partition asked me, and I nodded. The door ahead of me buzzed, and I pushed through it.

"This way, please," she said, and she led me to a small room off the main hallway. Opening the door, I was greeted by a tearful Gina. She hugged my neck, and we sat down.

"I thought you would never get here," she sobbed. "What took you so long?"

I rolled my eyes. "I tried to find the hospital following Mike's directions. I took Rosedale off the freeway, but the road was torn up and I couldn't find any sign for a hospital. Finally I saw what looked like a hospital and stopped there. It turned out to be a maternity hospital, but they gave me directions here."

Shelly's cell phone speed dialed my phone again, and once again got no answer. "Why doesn't he answer his cell phone?" she asked, panic in her voice. Tears ran down her face and Missy's. She sped down Old Betsy Road toward the freeway.

She dialed her office. "Patricia, any luck on finding out where Matt's been taken?" she asked for the sixth time.

"Yes," the voice said this time. "They have taken him to Harris Methodist Hospital."

"Thank you!" Shelly answered.

"Shelly, we want you to know that everyone here is praying for Matt," Patricia said.

"Thank you, Patricia," Shelly repeated, and hung up.

"I'm going to shoot that husband of mine for not turning on his cell phone," she muttered.

The phone book turned out to be useless, but I gripped it nevertheless. I wanted to do something, anything, to help the situation along. Instead, I was in the position that all parents dread, being helpless while your child is in desperate straits. Over the past few years, as my son, and then my daughter, had left academy for college and they were less and less under our control, I realized there comes a time when the only thing parents can do for their children is pray. I was in that situation now.

I sat on the leather couch in the small family waiting room outside of the ER. Gina sat across from me, and we talked quietly. The hospital chaplain, a small, kind Korean-American man, supported us, and left regularly to see if he could get any updates. Right now, the only news he could give us was that there was no news. Matt had arrived via CareFlite helicopter, we knew, and they were working on him. The only questions were what had delayed the trip to the hospital and how was he doing now?

The door opened and the chaplain led Shelly and Missy in, their faces red from crying. Shelly hugged me, and Missy hugged Gina, then Shelly pulled away and punched me on the chest for not having my cell phone with me. I showed them the phone book, and they laughed.

Mike finally arrived and joined us in the small room. He relayed to Shelly and Missy what had happened at the accident. He seemed a lot calmer than he had been at the crash site. Shelly put out her hand and placed it on Mike's arm.

"We are so glad you were there when the accident happened, Mike," she said.

Mike hung his head. "Cassie said the accident was my fault. That if I hadn't been in the next car, Matt wouldn't have crashed." Cassie was his on-again, off-again girlfriend.

Shelly and I looked at each other. *What a horrible thing to say.*

"Mike, if you hadn't been there, Matt would probably have died," Shelly told him. "You positioned him so he could breathe. God put you there." She stood and gave him a hug.

The door opened again, and Bob and Bev Mendenhall came in. Bob was my fellow professor in the communication department. Technically, he was my superior, but he was more a friend than a boss. Everyone hugged.

"How did you hear about the accident?" I asked. I had thought about calling my radio station and putting out a prayer request, but—once again—I remembered that I didn't have my cell phone.

"I called the station," Gina offered.

"Ben at KJCR called me," Bob said. "Then I think he called the university switchboard. You have people all over school praying for Matt." He put his hand on my shoulder.

"The first thing I did when I heard the news was call Jeff to make sure he was OK," Bob said. Jeff was Bob's son and a good friend and classmate of Matt's.

"I just want you to know not to worry about your classes," Bob said. "I can cover for you for however long this takes."

I nodded. I was hearing his words, but my mind was in search of other words—those of the emergency-room doctor.

"I just want to know that his vital signs are stable, that he's out of immediate danger," I thought aloud. "Then maybe I can take a breath."

As if in response to my spoken request, a rap came on the door, and a woman in blue scrubs and a stethoscope poked her head in the doorway.

"Mr. and Mrs. Robinson?" she asked. "I am the emergency-room liaison nurse working with your son. I came back to give you an update on Matthew." Shelly and I stood to hear the news.

"Matt vomited and aspirated a lot of emesis at the accident. The paramedics had a hard time intubating him so he could breathe. We almost lost him several times there, and his blood pressure dropped off the scale."

"But are his vital signs stable?" I asked breathlessly.

The nurse nodded. "He's stable. He hit his head pretty hard, and that's going to take some work and time to heal. But we are cleaning him up right now, and in a few minutes we will give you a chance to come back and see him. Family only, though."

Not My Son, Lord!

Stable. I had fixated on the word, somehow believing that if they could stabilize him, everything else would be OK. I sunk into my chair, the tension in my neck and shoulders relieved for at least a moment. For now my son would live.

It sounded like a case of his having difficulty breathing, which had been resolved, and maybe a concussion. Even now my wishful thinking told me that a couple of days in the hospital would probably result in his return home, with everything back to normal. What I didn't know was that *normal* was a state that would elude us for years to come.

A few minutes later Shelly, Missy, and I were allowed to see Matt. In a treatment room in the trauma center, Matt was stretched out on his back, his shirt and pants cut away, a green sheet covering his body. A nurse worked on his right hand, sewing up gashes across the knuckles. Another cleaned up his face, while a third adjusted medical equipment at his head. A half-dozen tubes ran across Matt's chest, up his chin, into his mouth and down his throat. He looked as if he would choke on them if he were awake. Blood had coagulated at the entrance of each ear, and a slight trickle of blood still ran from his nose.

Shelly started to cry, and I felt my knees start to buckle. This was no slight bump on the head. Both eyes were swollen shut, the sockets completely hidden by the puffy tissue that covered them.

I tried to put on a clinical air. Years before, working in hospital public relations, I had taken many pictures in ER and surgery. I had learned to deal with blood by focusing on the technical aspects, things like shutter speed and the angle of the camera shot. It had gotten me through many otherwise gruesome incidents. I focused on what the technicians were doing.

"How does his hand look?" I asked the person sewing up his knuckles.

"Amazingly well," he said. "It looks bad, but there are no broken bones." I watched as the metal needle disappeared into my son's skin and reappeared out the other side, pulling the cuts closed. I turned my attention to his forehead.

The medical personnel had done a good job of cleaning the blood away from Matt's face, but it was still evident that he had been through tremendous trauma. Both eyebrows had savage slashes across the center of them.

"Those look pretty deep," I said, watching a nurse manipulate the open skin around the left eyebrow.

"Yeah," he said casually. "This one is open all the way to the brain."

"Sir? Sir?" I heard a woman's voice ask next. "Would you come with me, please?" A nurse grabbed my arm and walked me over to a chair outside the treatment room. I didn't realize that I looked woozy. I blinked a couple of times and sat down.

The nurse brought me a soda and ordered me to sit there for a few minutes. I sat there, numb to what was happening around me. *It wasn't happening. It couldn't be happening. Just a couple of hours ago, Matt had been preparing to fly to Portland. Friends there were still waiting for his flight to arrive. Now he was a couple of breaths away from death.*

A physician in a white lab coat stepped forward and introduced himself to Shelly. I put my soda down and stood to join them.

"I am Bill Morgan, your son's trauma physician. I want to show you an X-ray and give you an idea of what we are facing." We stood together, looking at a gray X-ray film stuck onto a white illuminator.

"Matthew sustained a severe blow to the frontal sinus areas on both sides, with somewhat a more severe impact on the left side." Dr. Morgan circled with the tip of his pen to indicate the regions above the eye sockets. "The facial bones appear to be broken on both sides, but there is no serious arterial bleeding in this area. There is blunt trauma to the brain, however."

He turned away from the X-ray and faced us. "It appears his head hit something solid in the car, whether it was the windshield, the steering wheel, or something else. The brain sits in the skull like Jell-O in a bowl." He cupped his hands to illustrate. "You bang the edge of that bowl against something, and that Jell-O is going to slosh back and forth against the side. When that happens, you are going to get a lot of bruising, or even bleeding. That's what we are dealing with."

Dr. Morgan turned back to the X-ray. "In these cases, one of the things we are concerned with is pressure from swelling inside the brain cavity. We will need to drill a hole into the top of Matt's skull and place a monitor there to keep track of pressure. If he gets too much pressure in that intercranial cavity, it could cause more trauma—or even kill him."

"The other concern we have is this." The physician circled the left sinus area. "This fracture opened up the brain to the outside world. This could result in infection. We will be watching this wound very carefully."

"Dr. Morgan, what are the likely long-term effects of this injury?" Shelly asked.

"It's too early to be talking about long-term effects," he answered. "We just don't know. The Glasgow Coma Index measures the depth of comas with a score of three to fifteen, with three being the deepest coma. Matt was scored as a three."

The information was whizzing past me too fast for me to comprehend. I learned later that patients with a Glasgow Coma Score of three had a 10 percent chance of recovering with relatively normal function. Sometimes it is good not to know too much.

CHAPTER *one*

"But even that isn't my biggest concern at this time," Dr. Morgan continued. He pulled the head X-ray down and put one up showing Matt's chest. "This is."

His pen rose and circled a white cloudy area on both sides of the chest. "Apparently, Matt had eaten just before the accident and vomited at the crash. That vomit has gone back into his lungs. The paramedics had a difficult time intubating him at the crash site, and right now a respirator is necessary to keep him breathing. It will be difficult to get this foreign matter out of his lungs. But until we do, there is a high probability of Matt getting pneumonia."

I looked over at Shelly, who seemed worried but surprisingly composed. Her years as a registered nurse gave her a knowledge base I didn't have—but I also knew that the entire ballgame changes when the patient is your own child. "Thank you, Dr. Morgan, for all you have done to get him this far, and what you continue to do," she said.

The import of what was being said staggered me, and I was having a difficult time grasping everything. But still I insisted in finding something positive in all the bad news.

"Well, it could be a lot worse," I said hopefully. "I mean, there are no broken bones or damage to internal organs." My voice trailed off as I realized how foolish I sounded.

Dr. Morgan looked at me and blinked. "It could be a lot better," he said sharply. "He could have been at home sitting safely on the couch. Instead he's here on a gurney being worked on by a trauma team and being kept alive by a respirator."

As Dr. Morgan walked away, I desperately tried to grasp some semblance of composure. My concept of a predictable future and a stable environment had been ripped away in an instant. Now my family and I headed to the waiting room of the trauma intensive care unit (TICU) where Matt would be transferred in coming hours.

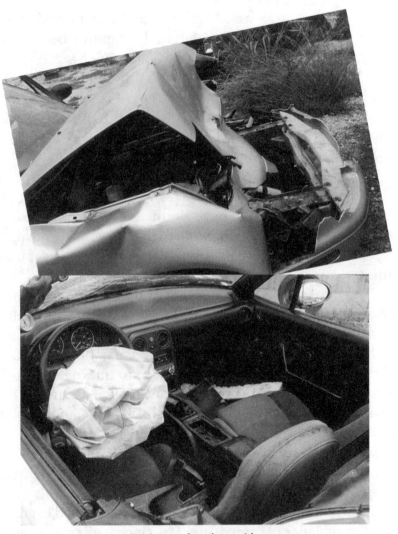

Matt's car after the accident

CHAPTER two

We left the emergency waiting room at about 6:00 P.M., three and a half hours after the accident. Tammy Tubbs, a nurse's aide at Harris, led us to the trauma ICU waiting room. Tammy was Gina's roommate and, of course, knew Matt quite well from his many visits to Gina's apartment. I didn't know Tammy, but her warm, caring, helpfulness would endear her to us over the weeks to come. Without her, we would have been frequently lost in the immense building—and organization—known as Harris Methodist Hospital.

Tammy led Shelly, Missy, and me, and the growing entourage of concerned friends, through the confusing hallways and over to the elevators that led to TICU. By now, I had fallen into a silent stupor, numb beyond belief. Matt was alive, thank God, but beyond that, none of us had a clue what would happen.

The TICU waiting room was a world unto itself, in more ways than one, we would learn over the coming weeks. With its dark paneling, green carpeting, and relatively uncomfortable padded chairs, it appeared like pretty much any other waiting room in the hospital. Two exceptions made it obvious that it was not. First, a small kitchen adjoined the lounge area. In it were a telephone, a sink, a small table and chairs, a microwave, vending machines, and a refrigerator. We learned as time went on that the refrigerator was always stocked with food, not through the courtesy of the hospital but through the ongoing compassion of caring friends and the other families who shared our plight.

The second fact that made the TICU unique was that the nature of the patient's injuries in TICU determined how the waiting room was used. Rather than waiting for a few hours for a surgical procedure or examination to be completed, with a doctor's verdict offering some closure, the families who occupied the TICU waiting room waited for results that might take days, weeks, even months to come to them. The waiting room was a campsite for the families of the critically ill.

When we arrived, three other families had already staked out their campsites, a fact made obvious from the blankets laid across chairs or on floors, the stacks of bags and coats, and the huddled groups caught in quiet, desperate conversation. The Mitchells* were the senior family there and had staked out the most private area of the L-shaped room, beyond the kitchenette in the southeast corner. They were there because their twenty-year-old son had been thrown from a car traveling at full speed. He lay in TICU in a coma.

The Hubbards* were nearest to them, camping just north of their site. This brother and sister had flown from Ohio to be with their father as he lay dying. They had come expecting it to be over in a few days. It had been three weeks so far.

The third family—the Gomezes*—staked out the northwest corner of the room. Their little daughter was struggling to survive after she had been hit by a car while riding

---

* Not their real names.

her bicycle. Until we arrived, they had been considered the newcomers. I learned with time that each family that arrived and settled in endured several phases of the waiting/hoping/grieving process. The first was a state of confusion, and we were there. When the visitors left and the grinding process of waiting began for us, the veteran families would come to us, introduce themselves, give us an orientation of the area, and make us feel part of the community that existed in this tenuous state.

Phones were scattered around the room and, as we were to learn, provided our single most significant source of information. The families of the TICU waiting room assumed responsibility for answering the phones, regardless of whom it might be for. Phone calls signaled connection with the outside world, such as calls from family and friends, asking for updates and passing on prayers and well wishes. They represented calls from the TICU staff, letting us know when we could go back and visit the patient. And they signaled ongoing news from medical personnel, updating us on the progress—however small—our loved one had exhibited. In any case, any news was good news. Our lives were lived in baby steps, one minuscule improvement at a time.

The TICU staff was incredible, we were to learn. They allowed visitors in to see Matt any time, day or night. That flexibility came in exceptionally handy for Matt's friends, many of whom were restaurant servers and didn't get off work until midnight or later. Matt was asleep in a coma 24/7, and the bright lights were always on, so the hours of visiting in TICU didn't affect him at all. Each nurse had two patients and kept close watch over them. Matt would have been thrilled to see his nurses: two were beautiful blond women about Matt's age; the third, who we met later, was a male nurse named Sergio who loved fast cars.

Not My Son, Lord!

Once we arrived in the TICU waiting room, it was hours until Matt would be transferred and fixed up with tubes and monitors and we would be able to see him again. In the meantime, the phone calls and the visitors began to roll in.

Gina, Mike, and Shelly all had their cell phones busy, and the TICU phone began ringing for us as well. Calls came in from California, Indiana, Colorado, Michigan, Washington, Idaho, and a dozen other states. The word had gone out like wildfire: The Robinson family was hurting, and we needed everyone's prayers and support. I heard from each member of my extended family, Matt's academy and college friends, a number of fellow faculty from SWAU, and the pastoral staff at Keene Seventh-day Adventist Church. Shelly's corporate bosses came to see if we needed anything. We learned that prayer groups had sprung up everywhere, including Keene Church, the university, Matt's doctor's office, and Wedgewood Baptist Church in Fort Worth, where a teenager had shot several at prayer meeting the year before.

The Olive Garden restaurant, where Matt had worked, demonstrated a love and support that surprised us. Matt had always made friends easily, and it was apparent that he had scores of friends at Olive Garden, many of whom he had touched in a significant way. Later they provided meal after sumptuous meal to us free of charge as we waited for news of Matt's recovery.

After about an hour of waiting for Matt to arrive, someone suggested that we form a circle and pray for his recovery. As we gathered the well-wishers together, I counted sixteen of Matt's friends who had come to support us during this trying time. My eyes scanned their young faces, and I found a new respect for my young son. He had touched more people than I could have imagined.

We took turns praying, and then I looked up and around the room. The Mitchells and the Hubbards had stopped their talking to listen and watch the group of concerned friends who stood in a circle in the middle of the room. These people who had seen so much tragedy in their own lives identified with the trauma that we were experiencing. A bond began to grow.

We continued to answer phone calls until 10:00 P.M., when we were finally told that visiting could begin, two at a time. Bill Kilgore, who had been Matt's favorite religion professor at Southwestern, offered to anoint Matt, and we got permission for him to go in with Shelly and me, Missy, Mike, and Gina.

The big wooden doors that kept us out of the TICU ward opened with a loud electronic click, and the six of us entered Matt's area for the first time. We were instructed to wash our hands at a small sink by the entrance. We took turns washing, then entered the TICU. A nurse sat at a circular workstation in the center of the unit, with TICU patients occupying glass-enclosed units on three sides of the desk. Matt was in bed four.

We filed into his room and were immediately overwhelmed by the seriousness of Matt's condition. He wore a neck brace, and an oxygen mask covered his nose and mouth. A gigantic metal tree full of monitors and other equipment stood behind Matt's head. A blue bellows over Matt's left shoulder rose and fell with his breathing. A tube, known as a central line, ran across his chest and presumably into his body beneath the sheet. Bandages covered the stitches in his right hand. His eyes were swollen beyond recognition, and stitches ran across both eyebrows. Traces of dried blood still clung to the entrances of his nose and his ears, and tubes still filled his mouth. The newest addition was a foam cup that was taped to the top of a shaved portion of his head. I knew that the cup covered the metal bolt and monitor they had inserted into his brain cavity.

Not My Son, Lord!

Missy grabbed my arm as we quietly walked into his room. I knew that the idea of anointing Matt was bothering her. Frequently we improperly associate anointing someone with giving up on them, a process similar to the ritual of last rites. I knew that it really meant that we were calling on a special portion of God's healing power, and I was grateful for that.

Pastor Kilgore stood at Matt's head, and the rest of us gathered around the bed.

"First, I want Matt to know who is here and why we are here," Pastor Kilgore said. "Matt, this is Pastor Kilgore, and we are here to anoint you and put you in God's protective power." He then asked for each of us to tell Matt who we were.

Pastor Kilgore continued. "We come here today because the Bible, in James chapter 5, says that if any of us is sick we should call the elders to pray over him and anoint him with oil in the name of the Lord. The Bible promises that the Lord will raise him up.

"Oil is used for a lot of different things in the Christian church," Pastor Kilgore explained as he put a drop on each of our hands. "In this situation, we are calling on God to raise Matt up. That can come right away, with a miraculous healing. It can come later on. Or it can come at the resurrection."

Pastor Kilgore looked around the circle. "I'd like to know if any of you have a favorite verse you would like to share."

Shelly spoke up first. "My favorite one is in Romans 8: 'I am convinced that neither death nor life, neither angels nor demons, neither the present nor the future, nor any powers, neither height nor depth, nor anything else in creation, will be able to separate us from the love of God that is in Christ Jesus our Lord.'"

Just as in every other time I heard that verse, I felt a surge of optimism come through me. Then Gina spoke up.

"My favorite verse is Psalm 37:4: 'Trust in the Lord and He will give you the desires of your heart.' I think that promise is very appropriate for us to claim right now." She looked around the circle. "We desire Matt's healing, so we need to trust God." The rest of us nodded silently.

After Gina's verse, Pastor Kilgore had the six of us kneel around Matt's bed and pray. Then we stood and he dripped the oil just above the stitched and bloodied eyebrows and the puffed eyes of my son.

"This oil symbolizes the fact that we are putting Matt in God's hands," he said. We looked at each other solemnly, hugged, and left the room.

The TICU allowed others to come in and see Matt that evening. Two by two, the other friends filed into the TICU room to see him.

About eleven o'clock Missy came to Shelly and me. "I haven't eaten anything since breakfast," she said. "Is it OK if I go out with several of my friends and get something to eat?" We nodded, not realizing that Missy didn't have any money, but then, we didn't have any either. We discovered later that Pastor Kilgore had given Missy and the others twenty dollars.

Shelly and I sat in the TICU waiting room, unsure of what to do. The number of friends and well-wishers started to diminish as the hours got later, but we wanted to be close in case something new developed. Finally, Shelly spoke up: "We need to keep our health up. Let's go home and get some sleep."

I stared at the wall and exhaled slowly. "Tell you what," I said. "Let's both sleep at home tonight. Tomorrow night I will come and stay the night."

Not My Son, Lord!

She agreed—but with the stipulation that she stay the second night.

We ended up leaving Harris Methodist at 2:30 A.M. Mike refused to leave Matt's side and ended up staying in his room until 5:00 A.M., when the staff chased him out to do more X-rays. Missy had taken my pickup, so I rode home with Shelly. I found myself both wide awake and bone tired and knew that Shelly felt pretty much the same.

We didn't speak much on that ride home that night. We both knew that our lives had changed that afternoon, but we couldn't be sure what that change would include. What we didn't realize was that that ride home from Harris Methodist Hospital would be repeated countless times over the next two months.

That night Shelly took medication to help her sleep. I didn't, but probably should have. Lying there in the dark, staring at the ceiling while I listened to Shelly's breathing, I prayed. I had always believed that God and I had a special relationship, that He loved me and took care of me and my family. But now I partially understood how Jacob had felt when he wrestled with God.

Lord, I prayed, *I know that I have prayed for You to confront Matt with his own mortality, with his need for You.* And I realized that this confrontation included his whole family and all those friends who couldn't believe that something so severe and final could happen to one of their own.

Is it wrong for me to turn around and ask You to heal my son? I asked, weeping into my pillow. *I would gladly take his place in that bed. I just want him to know You.*

Nevertheless, I said finally, *I want Your will to be done. I want to turn everything over to You. I hurt so, but I want to turn that hurt over to You.*

Thank You, God, I breathed, and fell asleep.

That night, I dreamed—and God spoke to me. First, God showed me the story of Abraham and Isaac, where Abraham was told to offer up his son Isaac as a sacrifice to God. The dutiful servant, Abraham brought his son Isaac up to the top of Mount Moriah and then told him that God wished for him to be sacrificed. Isaac voluntarily lay on the altar and Abraham raised the knife. It was only because an angel held back Abraham's hand that Isaac was spared.

Then I dreamed of David and Jonathan. The son of Saul, Jonathan was nevertheless a follower of God and a righteous man. He was the heir to the throne of Israel, but it was in God's plan for David to take that throne and for Jonathan to step aside. One young man received the crown; the other died in battle. Both had been consistent with God's will.

Do you know what you ask when you say, "Thy will be done"? God asked me. *Are you ready to allow My will to happen, even if it does not agree with yours? Are you ready for Matt to die, to be bedridden or unable to function normally if that is My will?*

I awoke with those thoughts in my head. A new sobering insight hit me. God was God, after all, and He is all-knowing—but sometimes His ways are unknowable. Could I live with the results of His will? Could I honestly say, "Thy will be done"?

CHAPTER three

Shelly and I awoke early the next morning, a little more rested but still unsettled after the trauma of the previous day. We threw on our clothes, not worrying about breakfast, and were on the road again to the hospital in Shelly's Honda.

On the way, Shelly's cell phone chimed. She answered it while I drove. It was Dr. Morgan.

"Matt continues to have difficulty breathing," Dr. Morgan explained. "To help him with that, as well as to prevent as much infection as possible, we'd like your permission to perform a tracheotomy." The procedure consisted of cutting a slit in Matt's throat and inserting a tube into his trachea. Air would be pumped into his lungs via the tube, which was connected to a respirator. The advantage was that it bypassed the sinuses, which were badly damaged and now a source of infection.

Shelly didn't hesitate. "If that will help him, then yes, you have our permission," she said. She hung up and told me what they were planning on doing.

We arrived at Harris a few minutes later and parked in the garage across the street from the hospital. The day before, we had arrived in such a hurry that we had parked in the first wide place in the road we had found, and it was amazing that neither of us had received a parking ticket.

CHAPTER *three*

Now that we knew these visits would continue indefinitely, we needed to learn the necessary survival tactics.

When we arrived at 7:30 A.M., the TICU waiting room was relatively quiet. Mike sat there on the couch, his eyes closed. He looked tired, I thought, and I wondered how I looked.

"Hey, Mike," I said, and he opened his eyes. "You doing OK?"

He nodded. "I was in Matt's room till five. Then they chased me out to take him for some more X-rays."

"How is Matt doing?" Shelly asked.

"About the same. The unit is doing its shift change, so Matt can't have any visitors until they are done."

Shelly nodded. "That lets them keep patient confidentiality while giving report," she explained.

We talked to Mike for a while until the waiting room phone rang, and one of the Gomez family members answered it. "They are letting visitors in now," she said to the rest of us. The families in the waiting room lined up by twos to go see their loved ones. Shelly and I queued up, third in line. We dialed the TICU desk, identified ourselves, and asked if we could be let in to see Matt.

"Just a second," the voice said. Five seconds later, we heard a loud buzz at the end of the hall. The big double doors to TICU opened up, and we walked through. After washing our hands, we headed down to bed 4, where Matt lay, a prisoner to a dozen wires and tubes and the frailty of his own broken body.

Matt didn't look any better than he had the night before. In fact, if it were possible, he looked worse. His eyes and face were discolored and swollen. Wires ran from electrodes on his chest to a monitor behind his left shoulder. Tubes ran into his body to help him breathe, to feed him, and to empty his bladder. A new addition was a stomach tube that bypassed the injured mouth and head to insert food and fluid directly into the stomach.

Matt was totally dependent on the machines and the professionals that ran them for his life, and my illusions of a quick recovery were fading fast. In two ways, Matt did look better, however. The medical staff had taken great care to clean up Matt's appearance, and the dried blood that had caked his ears and nose was gone. In addition, the respiratory mask had been removed from his face, as it was now unnecessary. In its place, a tube the width of my thumb ran into the collar around his neck. I looked closer and saw how it entered his throat. His chest rose and fell in synch with the respirator that hissed behind him.

"Matt, it's Mom and Dad," Shelly said loudly, leaning forward and kissing him on the cheek and placing her hand on Matt's hand. I noticed that an IV ran into a vein in the back of that hand and made a mental note not to move it too much.

"How you doing, Matt?" I said to him, putting my hand on his shoulder. Our family had always been open about our affection for each other, and Matt was very physical. Even as a young adult, he did not hesitate to hug me or Shelly in public if he felt like it. I knew that physical contact would be important to him.

Shelly went on to talk to Matt as if he were awake, telling him what had happened to him and that he was in the hospital. I watched my wife talk to her son, my heart going out to both of them—in some ways more to Shelly because of the heartache that she was going through even as her son continued to sleep.

I stayed in Matt's room with him as Shelly left later to make some phone calls. I talked to Matt about who had come to visit him the night before, about the friends from Olive Garden that had been there, and those that I had met for the first time. I talked about what the doctor had told us the previous day and described the nurses and techs that came in and out of his room. I even described the room he was in. More than anything, I wanted him to hear my voice and know that he wasn't alone.

In the meantime, Shelly met with a Harris Methodist case worker in the TICU waiting room. The case worker asked about Matt's financial situation.

"Matt is no longer on our insurance because he is out of school," Shelly explained. "He is working full time as a server at a restaurant, but servers don't receive medical insurance or any other benefits."

"So he has no medical insurance at all," the case worker clarified.

"No."

"Well, Harris Methodist does have a fund for indigent patients," she said, pulling a form from her briefcase. "There's a charity organization that helps out with those who can't pay their bills for valid reasons. That could help with your expenses here. You will need to fill out this form and turn it in.

"In the meantime, you will have expenses from CareFlite for getting Matt here, the physicians involved, the laboratory, and radiology. You will need to make financial arrangements with them. Your best bet is to get Matt onto Medicaid as quickly as possible." She closed her briefcase and stood up. "We'll help you as much as we can. I'm sorry that your family has to go through this."

When I came out of TICU, the waiting room was a lot busier than when I had arrived. Gina and Missy had come back to the hospital, and they went in to see Matt. I sat down with Shelly, and she updated me on the visit with the case worker. Mike had disappeared to go get some breakfast. As we talked, more of Matt's friends appeared.

Not My Son, Lord!

After a short while, Gina and Missy returned, their faces beaming.

"The ICU nurse that was in there said that we should try to get Matt to squeeze our hand while we talked to him," Gina said. "And so we talked to him for a while and encouraged him to squeeze my hand. Sure enough, after a few minutes I got him to give my hand a little squeeze!"

The news hit us as our first small victory. Buried under layer after layer of damaged humanity, our son was still there and had tried to communicate with us. I grinned at Shelly, and she gave me a hug.

Lunchtime approached, and yet no one talked about being hungry. Suddenly two women appeared from down the hall, both carrying Olive Garden plastic bags loaded with food.

"Lunch is served, courtesy of Olive Garden," said a short, bubbly woman in her forties. She puffed her way down the hall from the elevator, bags in both hands. A young woman about Matt's age followed her.

The older woman walked up to us and set the bags down on the floor. "Hi," she said, putting her hand out to us. "I'm Carmen Nicholls. I am a good friend of Matt's."

She gestured behind her to the other woman. "This is my daughter Tasha. We both work with Matt."

She lifted the bags again. "Lunch is on Olive Garden," she said cheerfully.

I looked at the clock and realized that it was almost 1:00 P.M. and remembered that I hadn't had breakfast. Strangely, I still didn't have an appetite. Nevertheless, Shelly and I followed Carmen and Tasha into the waiting room kitchen, where they laid out our sumptuous lunch of fettuccine, cappellini, Caesar salad, and cheesecake. This was the first of many meals provided free by Olive Garden.

CHAPTER *three*

Later that afternoon, the medical staff stopped letting visitors in to see Matt, and for a long time, we didn't know why. As more and more of Matt's friends arrived, wanting to see him, they congregated in the waiting room, and we got an opportunity to meet them and get to know the many friends that Matt had made.

Finally, as afternoon became evening, Shelly and I got a call from Matt's nurse in TICU.

"Matt spiked a fever this afternoon," she explained. "We have spent the past couple of hours getting it under control, but you can come back and see him now."

Shelly and I went back to the unit. Matt had ice packs under each armpit and between his legs to bring his body temperature down. We never learned how high the fever had risen, but the ice gave us a general idea that it was pretty severe.

I put my hand on Matt's forehead and felt the heat rise from him. My heart welled, and I said to Shelly, "I wish I could change places with him."

We spent a few minutes with Matt, but knowing that others were in the lobby waiting to see him, we kept it short. David and Danielle went in to see him next, and then others. Carmen and Tasha had waited all afternoon to see him. They came out smiling.

That was Friday evening. I spent the night there at TICU, as Shelly and I had agreed, with Shelly scheduled to stay on Saturday night. Our main concern was that Matt would awaken from his coma sometime during the night, and we would not be there to help him in his confusion.

I watched the other waiting room families as they settled in for the night. The vinyl seats could be made into a bed if you got creative, circumventing the metal arm rest by bringing a bench or another chair to put your legs on. The unit provided blankets, and we had enough foresight to bring a pillow. I checked in on Matt one more time about eleven o'clock before I settled in for the night. At three I awoke and couldn't go back to sleep, so I buzzed the unit and they let me in to spend time with my son. His status hadn't changed; he lay sleeping on his back beneath the bright lights, tubes and wires connected to every part of his body, waiting for his body's cue to wake up.

Shelly came in the next morning, and I went home to shower and take a break. Sabbath afternoon, the radio station had a special event already planned. I used it as an opportunity to tell our listeners about what was happening in my family's life.

"Many of you have heard of the accident that happened to my son Matt on Thursday," I said into the microphone. "Some of you remember him from when he was a DJ here at the station last year and the year before. Many have called to ask how he is doing, to wish us well, and to tell us that he is in your prayers. I just wanted to take a few minutes this afternoon to ask for your continued prayers and to tell you how he is doing."

I continued by telling about the accident and that Matt was still in critical condition in ICU. I told that it was miraculous that he had survived this long and that I could see the effect of the many prayers for him. I answered several phone calls from listeners who had heard of the accident, several who said that their school, their church, or their prayer group was remembering him in their prayers.

Several hours later, I went off the air and walked to my office. One of the student staffers gave me a large manila envelope.

"A listener left it for you," she said. "He wouldn't leave his name."

I opened my office and sat down at my desk, unsealing the envelope.

CHAPTER *three*

Inside was a magazine article about traumatic brain injury, stating that the damage to the brain could cause the victim to lose all interest in religion, become mean and angry, and lose all inhibition.

I looked at it for a long minute, then tossed it into the trash.

CHAPTER four

As we talked with Dr. Morgan, the ICU nurses, and the other families camped in the TICU waiting room, one message began to sink in: The ordeal before us needed to be viewed as a marathon rather than a sprint. Shelly and I had been caught up in the hope that the struggle would be resolved in a matter of a few days—or a couple of weeks at most. Now we slowly accepted the fact that quick resolution was highly unlikely.

"The brain is the slowest organ in the body to heal," Dr. Morgan explained to us. "It will take lots of time; some of it here in the hospital, much of it elsewhere once Matt is discharged."

In any case, Shelly and I started making plans for our lives during this time while Matt was in the hospital. She and I worked full time; Missy was a full-time university student. Our superiors had been very patient with us and with our situation up to this point, but we agreed that we didn't want to push that patience more than was necessary.

I had skipped my classes on Friday but was back in the classroom teaching on Monday morning. Fortunately, my classes all met in the morning. In addition, my second job as radio station manager was covered by a competent staff that knew what needed to be done and could be counted on to do their jobs with a minimum of supervision. The biggest challenge I faced at KJCR was that our annual fundraising event was less than a month away. I would rely on my staff and prayer a great deal during this time.

Shelly headed back to her office. She had started a new job as manager just two weeks before Matt's accident. Now she had the double challenge of learning a new position as well as supporting a son in ICU.

We decided to alternate our visits to Harris Methodist. My schedule had the most flexibility, so I volunteered to be at the hospital in the afternoon. Shelly planned on getting off work as soon as possible in the evening and coming to the hospital to spend time with Matt. In addition, she would try to come in the morning as needed to meet with physicians who otherwise might not be available.

Monday afternoon, as I was leaving the university to go to Harris, Shelly gave me a call on my cell phone.

"Missy talked to me this morning," she told me. "She is concerned about having to juggle classes and visits to Matt. It is also hard for her to concentrate on her studies when she is surrounded by all the trauma and confusion going on about Matt. I told her it was OK for her not to go up to the hospital for a while."

I agreed that this was perfectly OK.

"In all that is going on," Shelly reminded me, "it is important to remember that we have two children, and they both need us."

I spent the afternoon with Matt, looking for any signs of improvement. The swelling on his face was receding very slowly, and the black coloration around the eyes was settling into a lighter purple. I held his hand and tried to get him to squeeze my fingers, and got a bit of a twitch from his hand. It was hard to tell if it had been intentional or just a muscle twitch, but I was grateful nonetheless. His coma hung like a wet blanket between me and my son, and I searched for any indication that he was still there, buried deep beneath his unconscious state.

Mike was there, as he usually was when he was not working. I sensed that he was getting sick from his lack of sleep and endless hours at the hospital. Sure enough, by Tuesday he was sick with a terrible cold and didn't come back for several days.

Shelly came as soon as she could get off work and shared some good news. Several people she worked with had heard the story of Matt's accident and wanted to help. Knowing that Matt had no insurance and that we probably had expenses that would be difficult to cover, numerous people had written checks to the "Matt Robinson Medical Fund," a bank account that didn't yet exist. On their prompting, we decided that we would open a new account.

In addition, Johnny Le, manager of the Olive Garden where Matt worked, came by that evening with a check for five hundred dollars to help with Matt's medical expenses. Several weeks later, a second check for five hundred dollars was presented to us by Olive Garden corporate office.

While others were in visiting Matt, Shelly and I talked that evening about Matt's financial position.

"I talked to Matt just two weeks ago and told him that we needed to find him some medical insurance," Shelly said bitterly. "I could just kick myself that I didn't follow through on that." I agreed that I would contact Sharon Leach, a friend who used to work at Southwestern and now worked with a hospital funding agency, to see if she could help get Matt on Medicaid.

CHAPTER *four*

I visited Sharon on Tuesday at her office in Fort Worth. She had heard about the accident and asked for an update on Matt. I told her how he was doing and the details of the accident.

Sharon told me that she didn't work directly with Medicaid, but took me across the hall to another agency that did. She introduced me to a kind woman who listened sympathetically to our story. She told me that in order to receive Medicaid, Matt would need to be accepted for Social Security, specifically SSI. The path of application was long and arduous, but they agreed to assist me free of charge, giving advice and answering questions along the way. I got the application forms and took them with me to fill out in the TICU waiting room.

Tuesday night Shelly was in the room with Matt when John Curnow, one of the pastors at our home church in Keene, came by to see Matt. The elderly pastor had been by earlier and had left a cartoon drawing of Snoopy he had made for Matt. Tonight he brought another.

"One never knows how much people hear and understand when they are in this situation," he said in his clipped British accent. "But even if Matt doesn't know that the drawings are here, they brighten up the room a bit, don't you think?"

Shelly smiled thinly. "He knows that they are here. He knows we are here."

Pastor Curnow looked at Shelly sympathetically. "Shelly, I hope you know that God didn't cause that accident. I hope you are not blaming Him for it."

"Oh no," Shelly replied. "We know that. We know that it was caused by Matt driving too fast and by a truck driver pulling out in front of him."

Pastor Curnow put his hand on Shelly's shoulder. "I just don't want you to be mad at God for something He didn't do."

Not My Son, Lord!

She shook her head. "I'm not mad. I'm feeling a lot of different things, but being mad at God is not one of them."

By the time I visited Matt on Wednesday, I realized that the TICU nurses were doing a fantastic job with his medical care, but his personal hygiene was apparently going to be left up to us. Matt was always a stickler for good grooming; he especially made sure that he shaved every day. I had jokingly suggested to him in the past that he grow a beard as I did on occasion, but he would not even consider it. Now it was very evident that Matt had not been shaved since the accident. I saw that if he was going to lose his six days of whiskers, I would need to be the one who took care of it.

So I took the initiative and asked the nurse for a razor. Because of all the sensitive electronic equipment operating around Matt, we were not allowed to use an electric razor, which was what Matt was accustomed to using. Instead, the nurse brought me a safety razor, a small basin, and some soap. I wet and lathered Matt's face, then carefully, tenderly, shaved his face with the small safety razor. The act was an opportunity for me to do something personal for my son that he couldn't do for himself, and I will always remember it. Even now, I choke up as I write about it. The only regret I have is that I couldn't shave his neck because of the collar that protected his spine and his tracheotomy.

After I told Shelly, Missy, and Gina about shaving Matt, they got involved in other areas of personal hygiene. Even though Matt had no food or water coming through his mouth for months to come, Shelly brushed his teeth for him using a special sponge on a stick that the unit provided. On several occasions, she also gave Matt his sponge bath to help

the nurses out. Missy and Gina spent weeks taking care of
Matt's skin, especially his hands and his exposed feet, which
were often cold.

Each day we noticed that Matt was receiving fewer and
fewer medications. On Thursday we got good news. Dr.
Morgan told Shelly that they were taking Matt off morphine. After the morphine was discontinued, it would
simply be a matter of the body deciding when it was ready
to wake up.

We called everyone we knew and asked them to pray. We
didn't know when Matt would wake up. We only prayed
that it would happen.

Friday morning, Shelly got the opportunity to go to the
hospital early. She entered TICU and turned the corner to
Matt's room just in time to see him sitting up, looking at
her, and smiling! Excited, she ran over and hugged him.
When she called me and told me the good news, it was all I
could do to concentrate on teaching my classes. My son was
out of his coma!

I finished up classes and got up to the hospital just about
lunchtime. Considering the good news, TICU bent the rules
and let Shelly, Missy, and I into the room with Matt all at
the same time. I rounded the corner and saw Matt's puffy,
discolored face with his eyes opened just slits through the
swelling. Shelly and Missy smiled from ear to ear. Missy
asked him a question that I didn't hear. Matt responded by
raising his left hand and shaking it from side to side, signaling "so-so."

Matt seemed to recognize his mother most of all. I wasn't
sure whether he recognized me, and none of us were sure
how much he was aware of what was going on. We told him
again and again what had happened, about the accident, the
helicopter flight, and where he was now. Time and again
he moved his lips as if trying to speak, and we had to

remind him that he couldn't speak because of the trach. Once he raised his hand to reach for the tube going into his throat, but the wires and tubes attached to his hand held it away from his throat.

"Honey," Shelly said to him, grasping his left arm. "You need to leave your tubes and wires alone. They are helping you get well."

I was concerned about how much he was aware of and how much he remembered, but I didn't think much beyond that. With the accident, we started reading more and more about traumatic brain injury, and our reading only made us realize that we knew very, very little about an incredibly complex, mysterious, frightening field. One thing I praised God for was the fact that I knew my son was no longer unconscious.

Our joy was short-lived, however. We told Gina and his other friends that Matt was awake and alert, and everyone wanted to come in to see him. By that evening, TICU once again shut down visitation because he had again developed a fever. The high fever not only threatened his health, it dropped him back into unconsciousness.

When the fever had not subsided by the next day, we cornered Dr. Morgan and asked about it.

"Matt is still a very sick boy," he told us. "We still have foreign matter in his lungs that we are having to suction out. In addition, there is still some intercranial bleeding going on. How he is today may not be how he is tomorrow or the next day.

"We're continuing to take pictures of his head and body as we think he needs them," he said. "But you have to remember that this is a long, long process."

Shelly looked at me, her face pinched in concern as Dr. Morgan left us.

CHAPTER *four*

"Good old Dr. Morgan," I said. "He always tells us exactly the way it is."

"Well, that's the way you want it, isn't it?" Shelly responded. "You don't want him to tell us things that aren't true."

"No," I said, agreeing. "No, I guess not."

This time, the fever was severe. In addition, CT scans of Matt's head showed that bleeding was continuing, and a lot of blood had pooled inside the brain cavity. We waited and prayed, prayed and waited. Our consolation was that we knew that scores, maybe hundreds, of other friends and family members were praying as well.

Two days later, Matt regained consciousness. But it was not the Matt we knew. He was disoriented, confused. He would seem to have a moment of clarity, recognizing people around him, then drift off into some other plane of consciousness.

Shelly and I spent a lot of time with him, in many cases because of his disorientation. When we were not there, the TICU team was forced to put Matt's arms in restraints, tying him down to keep him from pulling at the tubes and wires that sprouted all over his body. While Shelly and I were there, Matt allowed us to hold his hand and talk to him, which seemed to calm him down. Holding his hand also made it possible for us to keep his fingers off the tubes and wires that apparently itched and were uncomfortable. So we took turns spending long periods of time just sitting with Matt and trying to reduce his agitation.

By the end of the second weekend, Shelly and I were showing signs of wear and tear. Missy and Gina spent a lot of time with Matt while we got some rest. Mike was gone, sick with a cold. Even with the additional help, exhaustion became an everyday state of being. I would sit down in the waiting room, lay my head back on the marble windowsill behind the chairs, and within seconds fall asleep.

We continued to hear from doctors, nurses, and other people that we needed to brace ourselves for a marathon in Matt's recovery. And we had always accepted that verdict, consoling ourselves with the belief that at the end of the long road, we would have our son back, well and whole. Now we were coming to the realization that no one knew what Matt would be like when it was all over. Further, none of us had any control over what the final verdict would be.

CHAPTER five

Once again, my family and I were confronted with the realization that Matt's life—and his future—were out of our control. We could pray for his well-being, even for something specific, such as his being able to wake up. But in the end, if we truly believed that God loves us, that He loves Matt, the wisest thing would be to simply place Matt in God's hands and be willing to accept whatever God had in store for him.

Such trust may have been the wisest thing, but it was also the scariest and most difficult. If Matt died, would we be able to accept that his death was God's will and was the best thing that could happen for him? What if he awoke but could never speak again or couldn't function mentally? Were we prepared to have a previously healthy, intelligent, vibrant son live with us as an invalid for the rest of his life?

As we watched Matt struggle once again with fevers and disorientation, we noticed something else. He was vigorously using his left hand and arm, especially to pull on wires and tubes. He was even wiggling his left leg. But he didn't use either his right arm or leg. Nurses and Dr. Morgan regularly checked to see whether there was any response to stimulus on his right side, but both the arm and leg lay limp.

As we thought about it, it made sense. The greatest impact in the accident had been to Matt's left frontal lobe, and we knew that the left side of the brain controls the right side of the body. Dr. Morgan cautioned us to not draw any conclusions about Matt's future from what we saw in TICU, but we couldn't help but wonder—and fear—that Matt would be permanently paralyzed on his right side.

As we struggled with Matt's disorientation that week, we noticed that TICU was gradually removing some of the tubes and wires that were attached to Matt. Thursday marked two weeks since Matt's accident. I went in to see him after classes that afternoon and immediately noticed that he was doing better. The most obvious evidence of this was that he clearly recognized me. In days before, he seemed to know and appreciate his mom, but I was never sure if he could separate me from the countless other visitors he had. Today, however, he smiled when I came into the room and lifted his left hand as if to grasp mine.

That small action—like countless other minute victories we had experienced over the past two weeks and would continue to experience—gave me hope. He was getting better. I could see it now.

Dr. Morgan stepped into the room, carrying a clipboard.

"Hi there," he said, looking up from the chart.

"Hi, Dr. Morgan," I responded. "How do you think Matt is doing?"

Dr. Morgan smiled. "Well, let me ask you that same question. How do *you* think Matt is doing?"

I looked down at my son, who had turned his head to look at me. "I think he is doing very well."

"Well, I agree with you," Dr. Morgan said. "I think he is making good progress. So I suppose you want to know how much longer he is going to be here in TICU?"

I nodded.

"The last thing that is holding Matt back is the respirator. Matt needs to be able to breathe on his own before we transfer him to the step-down unit. We're going to try to make that step in the next day or so."

"And then he will begin speech and physical therapy?"

Dr. Morgan nodded. "When he is ready for it."

I felt a thrill run through my body, and after Dr. Morgan left, I quickly dialed Shelly's office number to tell her the good news. The next day, Friday, I came to the hospital and discovered that they had removed Matt from the respirator. Shelly joined me later that evening, and we spent some exciting, happy time with Matt. We shared with him the good news that he would be leaving TICU very soon.

Dr. Morgan stepped in while we were talking to Matt.

"Another bit of good news," he said. That got our attention quickly.

He pointed over his shoulder at another white-coated man who stood reading Matt's chart outside the room.

"That's Dr. Glenn Bixler. He's a rehabilitation doctor. He determines if Matt gets therapy and what kind of therapy he gets. He is a very, very smart guy, and one of the best in his field. Matt has progressed fast and far enough that Dr. Bixler has shown interest in Matt's case, and that is a very good sign."

Our attention shifted to the mysterious new physician who stood outside the room. As Dr. Morgan left us, we watched Dr. Bixler, hoping that we would have a chance to talk to him. After a few minutes, he did come in to join us. Like Dr. Morgan, he was about my age.

"Hello, I'm Dr. Glenn Bixler," he said, shaking our hands. "Well, I see our patient, Matt, got a bump on the head. He's doing fairly well, considering how bad the accident was."

I nodded. "A friend took pictures of the car afterward." I handed photos of the smashed Miata to Dr. Bixler. "His head hit the metal rim above the windshield," I explained, pointing to the photo.

Not My Son, Lord!

"Well, the only question I have is, How can a big guy like this fit into a little tiny car like that?" Dr. Bixler laughed at his own joke, and Shelly and I looked at each other. We needed this physician; we needed his expertise and the critical therapy that his presence signaled. Enduring his dry sense of humor was a small price to pay.

"OK, let me get a little bit of personal information about Matt and the family," Dr. Bixler said. "Matt is thirty years old?"

"No, he's twenty-three," Shelly corrected. "For some reason they got that wrong in the emergency room."

"In college?"

"Just graduated," I said. "He has a B.A. in communication."

"Smart kid," he said. "That is in his favor." Pause. "What about you, Shelly? What do you do?"

"I'm clinical coordinator for Community Hospice of Texas."

"Registered nurse?"

Shelly nodded.

"And you?" he said, looking up at me.

"I am a professor at Southwestern Adventist University," I said.

"So you're both Adventists? The whole family is Seventh-day Adventist?"

We nodded.

He leaned back. "Well I guess I need to give my little speech then." He looked seriously at Shelly and me.

"Medicine is a science and should be approached that way," he said. "A lot of people, especially Christians, get caught up in prayer and expect miracles to happen. I can't depend on or believe in miracles. I have to depend on hard facts, on science.

CHAPTER *five*

"What I am saying is this: Don't let your faith get in the way of Matt's healing."

Shelly and I looked at each other in silence. *What was he talking about?* Our faith was the only thing that gave us hope; that kept us from losing our sanity. Our faith was the foundation for Matt's healing. Our faith wouldn't be in the way of Matt's healing, because without it, he wouldn't *have* any healing.

The conversation with Dr. Bixler both encouraged us and frightened us. What lay in store for Matt?

Saturday the word was given that Matt would finally move out of TICU. We were elated, because not only did it signal a milestone in Matt's progress, it also meant that soon Matt would begin physical, occupational, and speech therapies. The staff of TICU asked us to bring Matt back to TICU when he was doing better. "We never see patients when they are well," one nurse said. "It means so much to see the work we have done have a successful conclusion."

The downside of moving to the third-floor medical-surgical ward was that Matt would have less attention from the nursing staff. Each nurse in TICU was responsible for only two patients; the nurses in 3-West were responsible for eight patients. The move was a vote of confidence that Matt needed less care. The question was, would he?

A few days after Matt moved to 3-West, I arrived to see him sleeping in a newly decorated room. Four girls from Olive Garden—"The Four Amigas" we called them—had decorated the room Hawaiian-style. Gold and yellow streamers ran across the ceiling in all directions. Brightly colored leis were hung from the walls and wrapped around some of the lamps. A cut-out hula girl leaned against one wall. Across from Matt's bed, a giant hand-made poster urged Matt to get well soon with photos from the four girls, as well as other friends and workers at Olive Garden.

The Four Amigas—as well as Carmen—took responsibility for keeping up Matt's morale and were constantly surprising us—and him—with unique ideas that kept us in stitches. One day they all showed up at Matt's bedside wearing glasses, fake noses, and mustaches. Another time they came and serenaded him with their rendition of "Lean on Me."

Mike—who was finally over his cold—was not to be outdone. He brought a life-sized stand-up poster of Britney Spears that Matt had had in their apartment and stood her in the room where Matt could see her, day or night. And knowing Matt's preference for a certain soft drink, he fashioned an IV bottle of Mountain Dew, hung it from the IV pole and taped the other end of it to Matt's arm. Unfortunately, the nursing staff on 3-West didn't see the humor of Matt's Mountain Dew IV, and it disappeared the day after he put it up.

When Matt first arrived on 3-West, he was able to respond positively or negatively to our questions by nodding or shaking his head. But the neck brace began to stiffen the joints and muscles in his neck, making it harder to move it. In addition, his lack of solid food made him weaker. We could see our robust son get thinner and thinner every day. Finally it got to the point where he could no longer shake his head yes or no. Carmen came up with a method for him to continue to communicate with us. He would hold up one finger for yes, and two fingers for no. We would often have to remind him what he needed to do to respond, and he often got confused, but the system worked. And from the time Matt learned the system until he went home, that was the main way that he communicated with his friends and family.

CHAPTER *five*

Those of us who had been with Matt regularly since the accident were familiar and comfortable with the way he looked and the fact that he often didn't seem to be aware of his surroundings or those in the room with him. We would talk to him as if he were listening regardless of whether he looked at us or not. When it came down to it, we had no evidence that he wasn't hearing what we were saying. It was just like when he was in his coma; there was no evidence that he didn't hear our words then either.

But others who had heard of the accident and came to visit him were shocked by what they saw. This tall, outgoing young man with the commanding presence was now curled up in a hospital bed, often unaware of those in the room with him. One faculty member who came to visit him stepped into the room and stopped six feet away from the bed. As he talked to us quietly, I noticed that he gradually backed farther and farther from Matt's bed until he was standing in the hallway. What might have been a longer visit ended prematurely.

I soon learned to give a little prep talk to those who were visiting Matt for the first time. Another of Matt's college friends had moved out of state but was in Texas on a visit and wanted to see Matt. I met him in the lobby and walked Jason up to Matt's room, talking to him in the elevator on the way up.

"I need to tell you that Matt has lost a lot of weight," I began. "He also may not look at you while you are there, but that doesn't mean he doesn't hear you. Just talk to him as you would normally."

Jason nodded confidently. We entered the room and I walked over to the far side of Matt's bed.

"Matt, Jason is here to see you," I said. "Jason, say Hi."

Jason quietly said Hi, but I could tell he was caught off guard by Matt's physical appearance. A normally outgoing person, Jason said very little during his visit, but simply stared at this twisted figure in the hospital bed. Later, however, he visited Matt at home several times while he was recovering.

The second week of November was designated Sharathon for KJCR. The annual fundraiser was the busiest time of the year for me. I was torn between my duty at the radio station and my desire to be with my son. I, along with the rest of my staff, dedicated our week's efforts to Matt and wore red armbands during the week to signal our solidarity in support for his recovery.

"I can't say thank you enough to those who have continued to pray for Matt's recovery and have shown their support," I said on the air. "You never know who is out there praying for you, but I do know that all those prayers make a world of difference. That's one of the blessings of Christian radio. We have the honor of spending time here in front of the microphone sharing a scripture or playing a Christian song. And I can share story after story about how a song has blessed someone who needed the message in that song at that particular time.

"We have no way of knowing which song is needed at any particular time. But the Holy Spirit knows—and works with us to make sure we play what is needed. That's the way prayer is too. The person we are praying for may need our prayers right at that moment, but we often don't know that until later. That's why the Bible tells us to pray without ceasing."

I got off the air and walked into the station lobby. Gina was holding a phone out to me.

"This is Glen Robinson," I said into the phone.

"Hi, I just wanted to tell you that what you said is so true," the woman's voice said. "You never know when you can be used by the Holy Spirit.

CHAPTER *five*

"My daughter and I were stuck in traffic on the freeway the day your son had that accident. We prayed for him there and decided to make that our ministry; to pray for those people whenever we passed an accident.

"Later, I was having some rough times," she said, her voice beginning to tremble. "You see, I am going through a divorce. And just the right song came over your station. It touched my heart so. I just knew that God cared and that I wasn't alone. It gave me courage to keep going.

"You see, what goes around, comes around."

As a thank-you to our listeners for their support, I and the rest of the staff at KJCR had decided to feature a free concert by contemporary Christian artist Al Denson. Mr. Denson sang on Saturday night at the Keene Adventist Church, just one night after we had closed our appeals for support at KJCR. I was privileged to introduce Al, and before I brought him onto the stage, I gave listeners an update on how Matt was doing. I told them the good news that he had been discharged from intensive care, and that he was beginning to use his right arm and leg again. The audience broke into applause. I had prayer with the group, and then I introduced Al Denson.

Mr. Denson came to the piano, obviously moved by both my personal involvement in Matt's situation and in the show of solidarity that the audience had demonstrated. It wasn't until later that I learned that he had been in a plane accident a few years before, and he had spent a long time recovering from serious injuries.

"I want to say a short prayer once again for both this Christian radio station and for this young man," Denson said. "God shows His love through miracles every day, and it is always a privilege to be part of one of those miracles."

He prayed and then treated the audience to a two-hour performance of his well-known songs, interspersed with praise songs that he invited the audience sing with him.

After the concert, I went up to Al Denson to thank him for his performance. "Make sure you let Matt know that we are praying for him," he told me.

As Matt settled in to his new ward, therapists began showing up to put Matt to work. But fever continued to plague him, and we found that Matt was sleeping more and more. Dr. Morgan explained that Matt's sleep center, located right in the center of the brain, had been bruised in the accident. Until that healed, Matt would sleep a great deal of the time and struggle to stay alert enough to do his therapy.

We had looked forward to Matt's getting the therapy he needed so he could get well and go home. But now there was no indication that he was making any progress. In fact, indications were that Matt was getting weaker. His arms began to fold up in front of him, and he began to curl into a fetal position. Even when awake, Matt was often unresponsive to the people around him.

We sensed that Matt was unaware of much that he was experiencing. In that regard, Matt's condition was harder on Missy, Shelly, and me than on Matt himself. Often I would drive home after seeing Matt, despondent after spending several hours with him and not once having him look at me or even squeeze my hand. Curled up and facing the wall, his young body looked more and more like something you would expect to find in a back room of a convalescent hospital.

In those situations, I had no one to turn to but God. I couldn't even lean on Shelly, for she struggled with the same fears and trials. God became a refuge for both of us, and the

CHAPTER *five*

long drive from Fort Worth to Cleburne would often be one long conversation with God for me.

After struggling with this discouraging situation for many days, I realized that Matt might be aware of more than we gave him credit for. I talked to Matt for a long time about incidental things going on in my life and realized that once again he was unresponsive to my attempts at communication. I then looked at his face and thought I recognized a look of discouragement.

"Matt," I said to him intensely. "We are in this together. What you are experiencing is temporary. You won't always be in the hospital. I want you to promise me that you won't give up. If you don't give up, I won't give up.

"Mom and I are here for you. We won't leave you here. We won't ship you off to some convalescent hospital. You are going to get better. But don't give up."

I looked for a response from Matt, but he didn't look at me.

"Matt, promise me you won't give up," I said, leaning close to him, the tears coming to my eyes. "Squeeze my hand if you promise."

I waited again for a response. There was still no look of recognition, but after a pause, his long, thin fingers squeezed my hand lightly.

I left his room later that evening, tears running down my face.

CHAPTER six

Matt had been eligible to leave TICU when he no longer needed the respirator to breathe. Now in his room in 3-West, he breathed fine on his own, but he still had the stump of a trach tube projecting from his throat. The short tube was left there for two reasons: to provide respirator assistance again if he regressed and to make the continued suctioning of fluid from his lungs possible.

Moving away from TICU resulted in more problems with Matt's lungs. At different times, he developed spots in both lungs that were the beginnings of pneumonia. They continued to fight this condition by suctioning as much of the fluid as they could and by dosing him with antibiotics.

Watching the process was very difficult for me. The technician would bring in a special suction pump, insert a plastic tube down Matt's trach tube, and suction out whatever phlegm or other viscous fluid that they could bring up. Matt would go from relaxed to near panic. He would cough and gag and act as if he were choking, his eyes bulging until the procedure ended.

The downside of the antibiotics was that they not only killed the bacteria in his lungs but also killed the natural flora that lived in Matt's mouth. The loss of his mouth flora resulted in Matt developing thrush. Treatment for the thick, white carpet of slime that lined his gums, tongue, and mouth was to scrub his mouth several times a day with the sponge equivalent of a toothbrush coated with a special medicine. As in TICU, the medical care was excellent in 3-West, but personal hygiene was, for the most part, left to his family.

And when we were there, we were glad to help him out. Gina and Missy continued to take care of Matt's skin. The dry air of the hospital made his skin crack, so it was important to protect his skin with lotion. When he was left for a long period of time in one position, we would make sure he got turned and then massage his skin to improve circulation. Because all food and fluid was traveling to his stomach via a stomach tube, his mouth dried out as well. Shelly brushed his teeth regularly, made sure he got his gums and tongue scrubbed for thrush, and moistened his lips. I made sure he was shaved. And we all helped by moving his arms and legs through their range of motion so that the joints wouldn't stiffen up.

Matt especially had trouble with his feet. During his entire stay in the hospital, his left leg and arm were continually active, especially if he was uncomfortable. In TICU, there had been no movement of his right arm and leg, and we worried that he would be paralyzed on his right side. Slowly, to our joy, he began to use that side again, at first only wiggling his toes slightly. Still, the right side was significantly weaker than the left, and for a long time, Matt refused to use his right hand or leg.

The nurses started having Matt sit up regularly, first in his hospital bed with the head raised. Later they put him in a high-backed wheelchair. Matt could not sit in a regular wheelchair because the weight of his neck collar pulled him over. Later his stiffness and weakness made it impossible even without the collar.

Not My Son, Lord!

So every day, the nurses would get him out of bed, awake or asleep, and strap him in his chair. He would try to sit straight, but would very soon slide to one side and begin to lean out of the chair, looking as if he were falling out. The chair featured a footrest, but he stood six feet, four inches, and the footrest was too high for him. Invariably his feet would hang loose. When they did, blood would drain to his feet. Regularly I would come and find his feet dangling beneath him, exposed to the cold air, swollen and blue.

One weekend morning I came to see him. He sat slumped over in his chair, spittle running from one corner of his mouth, and his right foot hanging limp toward the floor. I began to reposition him, when a nurse we referred to as "the drill sergeant" came in the door.

"Why don't you make him put his foot back up on the footrest?" she asked.

I shook my head. "He can't do it."

"Sure he can," she said, matter-of-factly. She then yelled, "MATT, PUT THAT FOOT BACK UP THERE!"

I jumped at her voice but saw Matt quickly pull his right foot back up into place on the footrest.

Despite being initially discouraged at Matt's lack of awareness, we were continually amazed and rewarded by the "small victories" that we lived to claim on Matt's behalf.

As Thanksgiving neared, Shelly and I were in Matt's room when my mother phoned. "Nanny," as she was called by her grandchildren, asked for an update on how Matt was doing. While I talked to her on the phone, Matt's eyes turned toward me talking on the phone.

"Let me talk to him," Nanny said.

"OK, but be aware that he can't respond," I told her. "Matt," I asked, holding the phone out. "Nanny wants to talk to you."

Immediately Matt reached out with his left hand, one of the most obvious gestures of awareness he had made in weeks. I gave him the phone receiver, and he pulled it up to his ear. He moved his lips as if to say hello, and I could hear his grandmother's voice talking to him over the phone. His eyes lighted up, and again and again he tried to speak. When it was obvious he was getting tired, we took the receiver away from him.

"Thanks," I told my mom. "That meant a lot to him."

"It meant a lot to me too," she said.

We had originally intended to fly the four of us to Nanny's house in California for Thanksgiving but, because of Matt's accident, decided to have Thanksgiving together in Matt's room. Since Matt was unable to eat any of the food we had prepared for Thanksgiving, we decided to surprise him with an early birthday gift. We bought a PlayStation 2 and surprised him with it on Thanksgiving Day. I attached it to his room TV and brought out Gran Turismo 3, a car-racing game I knew he loved.

After we ate our Thanksgiving dinner, Gina, Mike, David, and Danielle joined us in Matt's room. Mike placed Matt's hands on the controls. Even though his reaction time was very slow and he crashed quite a bit, Matt was able to get around the track. His friends were thrilled, and it was a joy to watch him concentrate on this game. They played one game and asked if he wanted to play another, but the effort of concentrating on just one game exhausted him. We asked him if he wanted to sleep, and Matt held up one finger for yes.

Matt had his good days and his bad days. On bad days, the fever would return, and he either slept or was unresponsive. We dreaded those days because we couldn't communicate with him. Worse yet, his therapists would come to do treatments, something we knew was necessary for him to improve. If he was asleep or did not respond to them, they would leave and go on to give therapy to the next patient. The fever and sleep-center problems Matt had kept him from getting the vital therapy he needed.

But on his good days, Matt not only responded to our conversations, he showed signs of having his old sense of humor back. Therapists would work with him, and even though he might not like what they made him do, he tried his hardest.

Matt had several excellent speech, physical, and occupational therapists. One OT in particular bears special mention. Jerry West showed sincere concern for Matt's progress and not only talked to us regularly about how he was doing and what we could do to help but tried a variety of treatments to get the best use out of Matt's hands and feet. Most important, she didn't let Matt shirk his work. She would cheerfully push him to do his absolute best, and kept him going, even if he was in a bad mood.

One day Shelly and I watched Jerry spend a rigorous OT session with Matt; we stood in awe of what progress they were making. The session completed, Jerry told us bye and headed out the door.

"Jerry's so good," I commented. "Matt, do you like Jerry?"

Matt held up two fingers, signaling no. Shelly and I laughed at how Matt responded to Jerry's tough love.

As Matt became more and more aware of his surroundings, I pointed out things that were going on outside, including the warm fall weather we were having. I sensed that Matt would like to go outside and asked him. He held up one finger for yes. The hospital had a patio below us, and occasionally we saw patients out there in the sun and fresh air.

CHAPTER *six*

Shelly found the charge nurse and asked, "We're wondering if we could take Matt outside for a few minutes," she asked.

The nurse shook her head. "There's too much risk of infection. But I can let you take him into the hall for a few minutes."

Shelly brought the information back to us. Disappointed, we decided that the hall was better than nothing.

"What do you think, Matt?" I asked him, as I stood behind his wheelchair. "Do you want to go into the hallway?" He responded by pointing in the direction of the door.

I grabbed the back of the wheelchair and pushed him toward the door.

"Here we go," I said, imitating a racing car. *"Rrrrrrumm, rrrum, rummm."* I shook the back of the chair, making it vibrate like a car.

Matt's eyes grew wide, a smile came onto his lips, and he pointed down the hall.

We took him down the hall to where the elevators were located. Near them were picture windows that allowed Matt to warm himself in the sun and look out into the big world that he missed. After about fifteen minutes, he began to tire, and we took him back to his room.

After that initial visit to the hallway, Matt constantly asked to get out of his room by pointing toward the door. When he was in bed, we had to get help getting him up and into his chair. Sometimes he was scheduled for therapy and he was not allowed to leave his room. But in all cases, we had to get permission before he went out into the hall.

The days of fall were ending, and as the leaves turned and fell, we knew that there would be few opportunities for him to get out of his room. One Sabbath afternoon, the warm fall air was especially inviting. Matt pointed for the door and his eyes were opened wide in anticipation. I saw Dr. Colquitt, Matt's infection-control physician, outside the door, going through his chart.

"Did you need to see Matt?" I asked. "Because we were going to take him out into the hall."

She looked up at me. "It's so beautiful outside. Why don't you take him out on the patio?"

I looked at her in surprise. "The charge nurse said we couldn't take him outside because of risk of infection."

Dr. Colquitt snorted. "Nonsense. He has more risk of infection in here than out there. Just a second." She motioned for us to wait while she walked over toward the nursing station.

Moments later she was back. "Just make sure he stays warm."

I told Shelly and Matt the good news. We left a sign on the door telling where we were in case any visitors came looking for Matt and headed for the elevators.

"How do we get out there?" I asked in the elevator.

"I think there is a recreation room off the unit one floor down," Shelly said.

The doors opened in front of us, and we tore out into the hallway, once again with me imitating the sounds of a car *"Vrooommm, Brummm-brummm"* and Matt grinning from ear to ear.

We found the second-floor unit, but the room was being used for a class. A dozen people in wheelchairs sat in a circle, tossing a big rubber ball to each other. We pushed our way into the room anyway. "Sorry. Excuse us," we said, as the class stopped and watched us wheel Matt through and out the door on the other side of the room.

The wide concrete floor was empty except for a couple of plastic chairs in the center and a pile of leaves that had collected nearby. Tall brick walls rose on either side of the

CHAPTER *six*

patio. But on the other two sides we could see the city of Fort Worth and the buildings that surrounded us.

After about half an hour, Missy and Gina joined us on the patio.

"Look at this!" Gina said, holding her hands out at her sides and walking toward Matt. He grinned from ear to ear. "What makes you so special that you get to go outside?"

"It's gorgeous, isn't it?" Shelly said. "But you can tell winter is coming. I am glad we got him out here while we could."

As wonderful as the fall air felt to me, I knew that Matt enjoyed it tremendously more. This was his first time out of the hospital building in more than a month. I determined that it would not be his last.

CHAPTER seven

"Have you thought about the future?" Dr. Bixler asked Shelly and me. "I mean, Matt will not be here forever. Even if he never gets any better, they won't let him stay here. He is, after all, a charity case."

Shelly and I looked at each other. Dr. Bixler was right. Harris Methodist had agreed to take Matt as a charity case. We knew if they hadn't, Matt's hospital bill would be in the hundreds of thousands of dollars. We couldn't expect the hospital to take care of Matt forever, nor would we want them to.

I had filled out the paperwork for Social Security in an effort to get Matt Medicaid coverage, but saw no progress on that front. The Social Security Administration was the biggest bureaucracy I had ever seen—or experienced—in my life.

"What are our options?" I asked Dr. Bixler while staring at Matt's prone body in the hospital bed.

"Well, the very best thing would be if you could get him into an inpatient rehabilitation facility. Baylor has a great facility in Dallas, one of the best in the country. They take a very limited number of charity cases there each year, based on potential of progress. If Matt can show that he is a good candidate for improvement, they might be willing to accept him."

"What if they don't?" Shelly asked. "Are there are other rehab facilities in the area?"

Dr. Bixler nodded. "There are others, such as Pate in Dallas and HealthSouth out of Fort Worth, but Baylor is the best."

"If he were your son," I said after a long pause, "and Baylor wouldn't take him on as a charity case, what would you do?" I stared at Dr. Bixler, looking for a reaction. There was none.

"Then I would sit down with Baylor and make some sort of arrangement. Second mortgage, something like that. I would get my son the best professional help I could."

I looked at the floor. Despite both Shelly and I being professionals, putting two children through college while I was pursuing a doctorate had already strained our pocketbooks to the breaking point. I wasn't sure how much money a second mortgage would free up, but it wouldn't be much. We would have to pray that Baylor saw potential in Matt and would give him a chance.

Baylor's representative visited Matt a couple days later while Shelly and I were at work. She got in touch two days later. "I'm sorry, but we have no charity slots available right now at Baylor," she told me over the phone.

"I see. Can you tell me if Matt's progress as a patient at Harris Methodist played any part in your decision?" I asked.

"We take that into consideration along with a lot of other factors," she replied. I understood. If Matt didn't show progress at Harris, he was unlikely to show progress at Baylor, and that would reflect on Baylor's overall success rate.

I paused and took a breath. "Understanding that he is an emancipated adult, we are still his parents and want to get the very best care possible for him. If we were to take out a second mortgage on our home, we might be able to find a little extra money. What would it take to get him into your program?"

"If you were paying cash instead of insurance, the minimum we could get him in for would be $20,000 a month for six months with a $35,000 deposit."

My heart sank. Apparently rehabilitation was intended only for the rich or the well-insured. There was no way we would even get the deposit together, much less pay for six months of therapy.

"Thank you very much," I said quietly and hung up the phone.

"What now?" I asked Dr. Bixler. "Baylor says no, and Pate and HealthSouth don't have openings."

"I think you should get in contact with this woman." Dr. Bixler handed me a business card. I read the name: R'Lene Mulkey.

"She is the local representative for the Texas Rehabilitation Commission. They have funds set aside for traumatic-brain-injury rehabilitation, both for comprehensive care and for vocational training. You probably won't see any assistance for a while—there is usually quite a waiting list—but at least you can get Matt on the list.

"In the meantime, I have heard rumblings that the hospital is interested in discharging Matt."

"Discharging him?" I echoed. "How can they do that? He's not well yet." I looked down at his bed-ridden form, still unable to eat, walk, or talk.

"Well or not, they look at progress. Is he continuing to make progress? Not much. So the service the hospital is doing here could well be done at a convalescent hospital. I think it's time we talked about institutionalizing Matt."

There was a moment's pause; then Shelly said the word that I was thinking.

"No. We won't put Matt in an institution. If it comes to it, we will take him home with us."

Dr. Bixler shook his head. "I would strongly advise against taking him home. Families are full of good intentions, but 90 percent of those who take a loved one home with them give up. It's just too hard."

"We can do it," I said. "Together we can take care of him." I looked over at Shelly and had one of those moments married couples share when you both know exactly what the other is thinking. *He's our son. We wouldn't consider anything else.*

As December wore on, case workers from the hospital came to see us more and more frequently, asking about Matt's progress, but saying between the lines that his days at the hospital were numbered. Matt continued to have good days and bad days, and for once I was glad for the bad days. When fever overtook Matt, discussion of discharging him disappeared. It was only when he was doing well that the case workers appeared and continued to threaten discharge.

Then I got a phone call from R'Lene Mulkey. "Mr. Robinson, I want to get the ball rolling on Matt getting the therapy he needs," she explained. "The first thing I need to do is open a file on him, and legally I am required to interview him."

That worried me. "I have to warn you that Matt can't talk, and in many situations he's not even responsive. He uses his fingers to communicate: One for yes and two for no. How communicative he is depends on how he feels that day."

"Then we will have to hope that he is having a good day. How does next Wednesday at two o'clock sound?"

Not My Son, Lord!

I was very stressed before the meeting. Matt had had another fever a few days before and was still very sluggish in responding to any conversations. I sat down to talk to him.

"Matt, there's a very important woman coming up to see you this afternoon," I explained. "She is from an organization called the Texas Rehabilitation Commission. In order for you to get back to the way you were, we need to get you physical and speech therapies when you leave the hospital. She is going to ask you some questions. I will make sure they are yes-or-no questions, and you need to answer them the best you can. Do you understand?"

Pause. Matt raised one finger, while staring straight ahead.

"Do you think you can sit through an interview? Or at least try?"

One finger.

R'Lene Mulkey arrived about a half hour later. I introduced R'Lene to Missy, who had been visiting, and then Missy excused herself.

"Matt, this is the woman I told you about," I said to Matt. "Can you raise a finger to tell her Hi?" Matt raised one finger, then shifted his eyes over to look at the woman who stood to the left side of his bed.

"Matt, it is very nice to meet you. Do you understand why I am here?" she asked. Matt raised one finger.

I slowly began to relax as I realized that Matt was going to do fine on the interview. The only hitch came when she asked him if he had any money and he said Yes. I raised an eyebrow when he agreed that he had more than a thousand dollars.

"That's news to me," I told her. "As far as I know, he doesn't have a dime."

The interview lasted about fifteen minutes. R'Lene got the information she needed and told me that Matt would be put on the waiting list.

"The funding is given from the state to the commission for a fiscal year," she explained. "When it is used up, it's gone until the next fiscal year, which begins July 1. There is a slight chance that Matt could get some funding before then, but more likely he will start his funding next July."

R'Lene looked around the room at the decorations, including the festive Hawaiian hula girl and trimmings left by The Four Amigas, the scores of get-well wishes posted on the wall facing Matt, and the Snoopy cartoons drawn by Pastor Curnow.

"Well, Matt, it looks like you have a lot of people who care about you," she said. "The love and prayers of your family and friends can do a lot to help you with your recovery."

"People's prayers have already done a great deal," I said. "Sometimes prayer and faith are all we have going for us. But Dr. Bixler warned us to not let our faith get in the way of his healing."

"Let me tell you about Dr. Bixler," R'Lene said frankly. "Dr. Bixler is an excellent doctor, one of the best, and very smart too. But we know as Christians that there is more than a physical battle going on here. There is a spiritual battle as well. And even though the doctors and nurses can do a lot to help Matt on the physical level, he needs that spiritual support as well."

She squeezed my arm. "Don't give up on your faith—or your prayers."

"I won't," I replied, as she stepped into the hall.

Efforts continued on all fronts to get Matt ready to be discharged. Robin, the speech therapist, surprised us by plugging Matt's trach. With no air coming through the tube, Matt was forced to breathe through his nose and mouth. She explained that the action was in anticipation of completely removing the tube. It also gave her a way of working with Matt on the first few steps toward talking again.

Robin was able to teach Matt to move his lips and say words silently. She even got him to blow air lightly through his lips. But she couldn't get him to use his vocal cords.

"Sometimes the throat and the vocal cords can be very sore if you haven't used them in a long time," she explained. "I will keep working with him."

Robin was also responsible for assessing Matt's ability to swallow. Until Matt could once again swallow success-fully, he would continue to need to be fed via a stomach tube. Any attempts to feed him or give him fluid before he was ready might result in more foreign matter in his lungs.

We watched the progress with Matt's swallowing and talking, hoping that one day we would come to the hospital and find that the trach had been removed. Instead, two days later we found that the tube had once again been unplugged and voice therapy had been discontinued. To our disap-pointment, we learned that Matt had developed phlegm in one of his lungs again, and they needed the trach to suction that lung.

Jerry, Matt's tough OT, continued to push Matt to do more and do better, regardless of the mood he was in. One morning we found Matt sitting on the side of his bed. The accomplishment was made possible only because two OTs supported him, one on either side, and Jerry sup-ported him from the back. Matt sat and smiled at us as we came in the doorway, his body propped up on three sides by three women, his grunting and straining OT team.

As Matt's discharge became more imminent, I grew increasingly nervous about what it would mean. The biggest worry I had were the fevers he continued to struggle with. Would we discharge Matt from the hospital, only to bring him back a few days later with a fever? If we did, how would we get him there, and would the hospital accept him back?

Several other medical professionals, including one of our own relatives, had said we were crazy for talking of taking Matt home. They agreed with Dr. Bixler that Matt should be put in a convalescent hospital. Their voices of concern made us ask ourselves if we were perhaps unrealistic to ever consider taking him home.

As I struggled with these thoughts, Dr. Colquitt came in to check on Matt while I was there. She must have seen the strain on my face.

"Are you doing OK?" she asked.

"I'm just worried about everything," I said to her. "What if he gets sick again? I am not sure we can handle it, but I know we can't—we *won't*—institutionalize him as Dr. Bixler suggests." I struggled hard to hold back tears. "They keep pressing us to discharge him, but how can they discharge him when he has these fevers every few days?"

"Don't worry," she said. "They need my signature to discharge him, and I won't sign until I know he is going to be OK." She smiled reassuringly from the other side of the bed.

As if by some signal, Matt's health suddenly got much better. He seemed alert and responsive, and there was no sign of fever. We arrived one morning, and Matt's trach tube had been completely removed. We asked Robin about it when she came in. She explained that not only was she going to step up his speech therapy, she was there to evaluate his ability to swallow. If he passed the swallowing test, he would soon be able to eat regular food.

We left that afternoon and went down to the hospital cafeteria, perhaps vicariously trying to swallow for Matt. We knew that taking care of him at home would be a lot easier if he passed the test. Not only that, but his quality of life would be better.

An hour later we went up to see how he did.

"Well, I tried a little water first," Robin said. "He did fine with that, so I tried some juice. He did fine with that as well, so then I got brave and decided to try some applesauce. He passed with flying colors!"

And so it was decided that Matt would be discharged within a couple of days. There remained one more hurdle, however. The nursing staff, skeptical of our ability to take care of Matt, required us to take care of him for one twenty-four-hour shift by ourselves before he could be discharged. They showed us how to mix his liquid food and feed it into his stomach tube. They showed us how to change his diapers, empty his catheter bag, and clean the catheter tube. They showed us how to turn him every hour so he didn't get pressure sores and how to use a hydraulic patient lift to transfer him to a wheelchair.

After twenty-seven years as a nurse, and experience as a nurse's aide before that, Shelly had an advantage over me, but I paid attention to the instructions and was determined to help as much as I could. Shelly and I shared the shifts until early the next morning—feeding, turning, and changing as were necessary. Gina, Missy, and Mike helped us the next day by coming in and giving us some time away.

CHAPTER *seven*

In addition, Nanny, my seventy-eight-year-old mother, with countless years of experience in nursing and taking care of a score of kids and grandkids, had flown in from California to help with the discharge as well. We had the support, we had the instruction, and we had made the decision to discharge. Most important, we had the continued prayers of hundreds of friends and family all over the world.

On December 13, Matt was discharged from Harris Methodist Hospital of Fort Worth to go home.

CHAPTER eight

I will never forget the trip home from Harris Methodist Hospital that day. We packed up all of Matt's belongings: the Britney Spears standup, the hula girl cutout on the wall, all his decorations, stuffed animals, cards, letters, and pictures sent by well-wishers. Shelly and I loaded all his "stuff" into the back of my small pickup. Then ambulance attendants came for Matt after he had been transferred to a gurney.

Matt has the ability to make friends even when he can't talk. Nurses lined up at his doorway when they wheeled him out, all wanting to wish him good luck and Godspeed. Just as with TICU, many asked for him to return and visit the unit when he was doing better. Six months later, we did just that. They were overjoyed to see how well he was doing, but—for better or for worse— he didn't remember any of the experience of being in the hospital.

And while he was moving down the hall, waving at the nurses, Matt's eyes were wide and bright, his mouth curved into a permanent grin. The grin didn't leave his face when they put him in the back of the ambulance, when they drove him the twenty-five miles south to our home in Cleburne, or when they rolled him up the front steps and into the house. He was home.

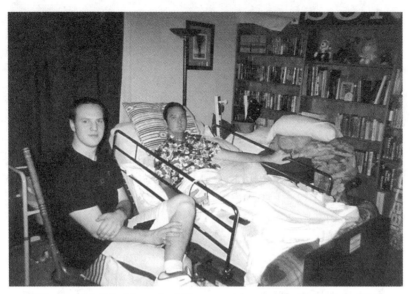

Mike and Matt in his makeshift room at home, late December, 2002

And despite the worries and the stress we may have felt about leaving the hospital, we were glad to have Matt home as well. It felt natural and perhaps gave us the first day of normalcy we had experienced in two months. It was hard not to believe that things were going to get better.

We knew that Matt was going to need a hospital bed. We also knew that he would need other equipment, such as a hydraulic lift to transfer his thin but still heavy body from the bed to his wheelchair. We knew that he would be getting visitors, and he would want to be in the middle of activity at home. So we transformed my study, located right by the front door, into Matt's bedroom.

The process of getting the room ready for him was therapeutic for us. We took on the project of fixing up the study with gusto, repainting and wallpapering to make the room bright and cheerful. We put curtains up over the picture window to give him privacy as well as to control the light for his daytime naps. And I installed new doors at one entrance and a privacy curtain at the other end of the room.

The training we received at Harris Methodist for Matt's care was not ignored. Matt was released from Harris the day after I turned in semester grades and had three weeks' vacation before the next semester. Shelly took primary responsibility for Matt in the evening, and I took care of him during the day. We alternated responsibility at night, with Missy stepping in to help us as well. Matt needed to be turned every two hours, his catheter needed to be emptied and cleaned, and he needed to be fed through his stomach tube. He also regularly needed bed baths and clean sheets. Although I had no training in it, once again I was grateful to do something for him to show how important he was to us.

And Nanny, my visiting mother, played a big part in helping with Matt. In fact, it was often difficult to hold her back. As much as has been said about a parent's love, a grandparent's love in some ways is just as strong.

We appreciated her support greatly but at the same time were concerned about her for several reasons. The most obvious reason was that she was seventy-eight years old, albeit a young seventy-eight years. In addition, just a few months before Matt's accident, she had been in an auto accident of her own, putting her in the hospital and taking the life of her second husband, Dyke. A short time after that, her brother had died of cancer. She had been on the plane going back to California from her brother's funeral in Oklahoma when she heard of Matt's accident. We were concerned that she hadn't had sufficient time to grieve and heal both physically and mentally from those two tragedies before she had come to Matt's aid. We appreciated her but watched her carefully.

CHAPTER *eight*

Matt came home on a Friday. When I checked on him the next morning, I found him lying on his right side, facing away from me. I crept around the foot of the bed, but saw that his eyes were open. He gave me a big smile when I walked up to him.

"Good morning," I said to him. "You're glad to be home, aren't you?"

He gave me a little nod. His neck was both gaining strength and loosening up since they had taken off his neck brace.

"The sun is shining outside," I said to him. "Do you want me to open the curtains?"

He slightly shook his head no. He gave me a contented look and exhaled slowly.

"You're just enjoying lying in bed, aren't you?" I said. He nodded, smiling.

"Good morning, Sleepyhead," Shelly said to him, coming up behind me. "How did you sleep? I thought we would try you on some food this morning. How does that sound?"

Matt nodded.

"We will need to feed you something pretty soft to begin with—yogurt, ramen, applesauce, maybe some scrambled eggs. What sounds good?"

Matt mouthed the word *eggs*.

"Eggs? OK, coming right up."

Shelly fixed us all some scrambled eggs, and I fed Matt. "Be careful not to give him too much at one time," she warned me, but he wolfed down the eggs as if he had been starving.

"You have lost a lot of weight," I told him. "I wonder how much."

"Let's get the scale. We can stand him up on it if you support him," Shelly suggested.

Shelly sat Matt on the side of the bed and let him get

comfortable, while I got the bathroom scale. Standing behind him to balance him, we got him to stand on the scale. It read 190. He had weighed 240 at the time of the accident. Even at six feet four inches, he could afford to lose a little weight, but fifty pounds, much of it muscle, was a bit extreme.

"Well, if he keeps eating like he did this morning, he will gain it back in no time," Nanny said, who had joined us. And he did. Matt's appetite became ravenous. Coupled with a limited amount of exercise in the first year, his weight went up to 280, then came back down when he became more physically active. Today it is once again 240.

While I went in the room to get Matt some clothes to wear, Shelly and Nanny decided to see if he could take some steps. One stood on each side of him and balanced him. Matt took two steps forward before having to sit back down. We were all amazed, considering that Matt had needed three OTs just to sit on the side of the bed just a short time before. This was the first time that Matt had stood in almost two months.

We became convinced that coming home was the best possible thing that could have happened to Matt. Not only did it help with his morale (and ours), it was less stressful, and he was willing to do more for his family. In addition, we discovered that much of the problem he had with fever was directly related to being in the hospital and exposed to other people's germs. After he came home, he never had a fever again.

After Matt's success with taking two steps, our challenge was to get him to take a few more steps each day. We had the hoist, and we made use of it, especially when Matt was tired. He still slept a lot each day, and his endurance still suffered. Often I would get him to take a few steps, and then have to rescue him with the wheelchair, which we always kept nearby.

CHAPTER *eight*

Because of Shelly's work with hospice, she had friends in the hospital-equipment business who charged her discount prices or, in some cases, nothing at all for the equipment we needed. One of the things she felt we would need was a walker with legs in the front and wheels in the back. The theory was that Matt would lean on the walker for balance, pushing it ahead of him as he walked along. He never got the walker to work the way it was supposed to. Instead, he would end up carrying it in front of him. We eventually set it aside, and we depended on a waist belt to help us balance him.

Matt was now able to hold up his head and so had moved from the high-backed wheelchair he used in the hospital to a regular one with leg supports. Although we encouraged him to walk for short distances—which were gradually getting farther—he still depended on the wheelchair for longer distances.

Eight days after he arrived home, Matt decided that he wanted to go to church. We took two vehicles to the Keene Adventist Church, with Matt riding in the front passenger seat of Shelly's Honda, and me loading his wheelchair into the back of my pickup and following behind. It took us quite a while to get from the parking lot to the sanctuary, mainly because so many people stopped to talk to Matt on the way. He smiled and nodded for all of the well-wishers' questions, but it was obvious that Matt didn't know many of the people who wished him well.

We pushed Matt's wheelchair through the crowd and to the back of the first section in the sanctuary, the area reserved for families with members who used wheelchairs. We had Matt stand up from the wheelchair and sit back down in the pew. That way we could support him better. As announcements were read from the pulpit, Pastor Don Baker, one of the many Keene pastors who had visited Matt in the hospital, welcomed the Robinson family—all of us—back to the Keene Church services. The sanctuary burst into spontaneous applause, and Shelly and I beamed.

It felt so good to be in church, not in a spirit of need and supplication, but in a spirit of thanksgiving. Our family was complete again, and all four of us (five counting Nanny) were in the house of the Lord to worship again. As the sermon started, I looked down the pew at Matt, who had already succumbed to fatigue and fallen asleep, leaning against Shelly's shoulders. *Let him sleep,* I thought, and I knew that God understood as well.

Matt was eating well now; in some cases, eating everything in sight. Our biggest concern, of course, was that Matt would inhale his food and get it into his lungs, leading back to pneumonia and another trip to the hospital. But Matt showed no hesitation in his ability to eat. To the contrary, he seemed to be in a race to catch up with all the eating he had missed while he was away. His marathon eating concerned me, especially as he started putting on weight. Dr. Bixler assured me at a later visit that increased eating and weight gain were common with brain injury and that we had larger issues to worry about.

It wasn't long before Matt was eating almost a normal diet. One interesting thing developed, however. Before the accident, he had not been fond of eggs and would never eat them when served at breakfast. After the accident, they became one of his favorite foods. Part of the reason for that may be that scrambled eggs were one of the first solid foods he was allowed to eat.

Even though Matt was walking a little and eating solid food, he was still unable to speak. We tried the techniques the speech therapist at Harris had taught us. We had Matt concentrate on blowing out candles, we had him put his hands on our vocal cords and try to make his do the same thing; we worked constantly with him.

Because Matt is a highly social person, I knew it was important to find a way to help him communicate. Wondering whether he still was able to type, I rolled Matt's wheelchair up to the computer console and typed: "Type something."

In response, he dragged his left index finger over the keys to type: "Something."

I had to adjust the sensitivity of the keyboard, because he could not take his fingers off the keys and the computer ended up typing *aaaaaaa* when he only wanted one *a*. It seemed like a good idea for allowing him to say what he needed to say beyond just yes or no. But we used it only once.

A few days later, I was pondering the problem of Matt's talking as I worked on a wire fence I was building around our backyard. With Matt and Nanny in the house, and more visitors coming around, we wanted our two dogs to remain in the backyard as much as possible. I had been working on the fence in my spare time for weeks and now had just about completed it.

I started thinking about the habit Matt had before the accident of clearing his throat constantly, something that I remembered that my father had done as well. As I thought about it, I realized that clearing the throat used the vocal cords, which Matt had not used since the accident. Further, clearing the throat was very similar to saying the *mmm* sound. If I could get Matt to do that, perhaps I could get him to say the word *Mom*.

I finished my work on the fence and came inside. Matt was sitting in my overstuffed chair in the living room, watching TV with Nanny.

Not My Son, Lord!

"Matt," I said. "I want you to try something. Do you remember before the accident how you used to clear your throat?"

He looked at me blankly, and I knew he wasn't sure what I was talking about.

"You used to do this a lot," I said, and made the *grrrrr* sound one makes clearing their throat. I took his hand and put it on my throat, letting him feel the vibration as I cleared my throat again. After a few times, I was able to get him to clear his throat as well.

"Now, let air out of your lungs and say the word *Mom*."

He pursed his lips and soundlessly mouthed the word *Mom*.

"Try it again," I said. "Remember how it felt to clear your throat."

We continued working on it for about half an hour. A little later on, Shelly came in the door, stopping by the house for lunch. I met her in the kitchen.

"Matt has a surprise for you," I said smiling.

"Oh he does, does he?" Shelly asked. She walked into the living room and saw Matt sitting in the overstuffed chair. "What surprise do you have for me?"

Matt looked up at her and smiled. "Hi, Mom," he whispered in a raspy voice.

Shelly's eyes grew large and she whooped in joy, hugging her son. "Oh, that's the best Christmas present you could ever give me!"

I look at that achievement as one of the greatest accomplishments in my life.

CHAPTER nine

A couple weeks after Matt came home, it was time for appointments with Drs. Morgan and Bixler in their offices. Dr. Bixler was surprised to see Matt roll through the door of his examination room in a wheelchair, alert and sitting straight and tall. It had been only a couple of weeks since he had last seen him, but the change was dramatic.

"Home must agree with him," he admitted.

Dr. Morgan's approach was more clinical. He asked us how Matt was doing with eating. By that time, Matt was eating sufficiently that we no longer needed to use his stomach tube.

"We're hoping you will be willing to take the tube out," we said, although we were a bit concerned about how difficult and invasive it would be to remove a tube that went through the abdominal wall and into the stomach.

Dr. Morgan nodded. "Seems like it is about time for that to happen." He had Matt lie flat on his back on the examination table, reached down, and pulled on the tube. The rubber tube came free with a pop. A bulb had held it in place. Dr. Morgan put a simple bandage over the opening, stating that it would heal closed within a few days.

Not My Son, Lord!

December 23 marked Matt's twenty-fourth birthday. We asked him where he would like to celebrate his birthday, and he said, "the Olive Garden." So we packed him up in the Honda and headed to Fort Worth. That evening happened to also be the Christmas party for Olive Garden staff. Before we could be settled into a table in the restaurant, several servers saw Matt and insisted that we join the staff party. The party was just winding down, but all of the servers were still there. They took turns coming up to Matt and asking him if he remembered them. Unfortunately, he remembered only about half of those who introduced themselves.

As had been the case when Matt was in the hospital, Olive Garden would not accept our payment for our food, but insisted we order whatever we wanted. Matt ordered his favorite: fettuccine Alfredo. Carmen was our server. Matt still needed assistance in eating; his hand strength and coordination was not good enough for him to feed himself, so we usually had to feed him. The Four Amigas took turns feeding him fettuccine, and as I watched one after another of the young attractive women feed my son, I could tell that Matt was thoroughly enjoying himself.

Christmas came and went; enjoyable because we were all at home, alive and safe. I had learned during the past two months that what we did as a family was far less important as the fact that we did it together. In addition, I learned to never again take the future for granted. God gives us one day at a time. There are no guarantees that our life will extend beyond that day, so it is important to learn to appreciate each day as it comes.

The weather turned cold right before Christmas and held on to its bite until after New Year's Day. Our two dogs,

CHAPTER *nine*

which were used to being inside the house, were continually begging to be let in. Shelly was worried about their bringing in germs that could make Matt sick in his weakened condition, so we tried to keep the dogs outside. We purchased a plastic igloo for them to sleep and stay in when it got cold. In addition, Shelly installed a heat lamp on our deck to keep them warm.

One morning when Matt and I were alone in the house, I had just finished feeding him and walked into the living room that was on the back side of the house. Through the window I saw flames shooting eight feet from the deck to the wooden eaves above it. Fire! I ran outside to see how bad it was. Fire about six feet across roared from the wooden deck against our living room and kitchen wall, with flames licking the roof above the deck. I dashed across the deck to the brick walkway behind the house and grabbed a water hose connected to a backyard faucet. I continued to spray the fire for nearly an hour before the sparks were gone and it had stopped smoldering.

When it was finally out, I took inventory of the damage. Two windows were cracked from the heat, and the paint above the fire was blackened. The deck itself had a big hole in it where the fire had burned the beams through. Apparently one of the dogs had bumped the heat lamp against something flammable, starting the fire.

I went in to check on Matt, whom I had been forced to leave on his own for nearly an hour. He sat contentedly in his hospital bed. I told him about the fire, grateful that I had walked into the living room in time to see the flames. Had the fire gotten into the attic space, it very likely would have spread to the rest of the house. I would have had a difficult time getting Matt out the door in time to save him. Once again, our guardian angels had saved us.

Not My Son, Lord!

Registration for school came at the beginning of January, which meant Missy and I needed to get back into the classroom. While sitting in the university library during registration, I saw Jean Thomas, a good friend and editor of the Southwestern Union *Record*. She told me that she desperately needed someone to write an article about answers to prayer, and she needed the article right away. I told her I could do it, and wrote an article about how my prayers for Matt to have a road-to-Damascus experience had been answered by his accident and that praying "Thy will be done" opened a whole new can of worms with God. I had learned, the hard way, to accept what God had for me. After the article was in print, numerous people at the Keene Church and at the university told me how they appreciated the article. What I didn't know was that the small article would reach far beyond its expected audience.

Nanny agreed to stay on for a few weeks and be with Matt during the day. We knew, however, that would be only a temporary fix. Shelly looked briefly at hiring someone to come in and be with Matt, but we worried whether we could afford it. She also contacted a woman she knew who took in people with disabilities who needed extended care. We dreaded the idea of Matt leaving home again, but we were running out of options.

Three weeks into the school year, we realized that Nanny had to get back to California. As much as we loved her, she needed to get back to the routine she was used to in her own home, and we needed to do the same. But we still hadn't come up with a solution for Matt. So once again we turned to prayer for an answer.

Shelly came to me a couple of days later. "Missy wants to drop out of school this semester," she told me. "She doesn't

CHAPTER *nine*

want anyone else taking care of Matt; she feels this is a problem we need to take care of as a family."

I thought about it long and hard. Missy was in her junior year. She was doing well in school, but I didn't want her to get behind and graduate late. I agreed with her that I would rather take care of Matt as a family instead of having someone from the outside come in to deal with him. In addition, Matt had moved beyond having to be fed

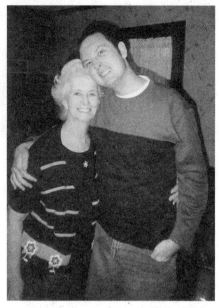

Matt with Nanny in February 2003

and diapered and, with a little help, could make it to the bathroom and take his own shower. Our biggest concern was his falling, and his sister was strong enough to help with that. I finally decided that she had come up with a workable solution.

I told Nanny a couple of days later, and she booked a flight for California. We will never be able to repay Nanny for her help and support during this trying time, but we were glad she was able to get back to her own home for the sake of her health and sanity.

Missy's sacrifice of a semester of school seemed to be the logical answer for our problem, but it was not as easy a solution as it appeared. Matt was used to being the older brother, just as Missy was used to being the younger sister, and they had accepted and embraced their roles in their years together. Now, in a sense, their roles were reversed. Missy had to learn to tell Matt what to do and to depend on herself when Matt leaned on her for support, instead of the other way around.

Matt's regained ability to speak opened up a Pandora's box of questions and issues that we hadn't known existed. We continued to learn about traumatic brain injury, but by now the learning was firsthand. The first thing we learned was that a large chunk of Matt's memory—from almost a year before the accident until the present—was totally gone. At first he insisted that we were in Idaho, where we had lived four years before, and continued to mention friends from academy that he hadn't seen in years. Later, he assumed that he was in Seattle, where he had lived for two years before coming to Texas. It took us quite a while to convince him that he was no longer in school and eventually had to show him his diploma to prove our point.

He believed he still lived in the loft, the apartment where he and Mike had been roommates for several months before he moved back home. He didn't remember certain people from his past and present, including a former girlfriend named Cindy that he had had a traumatic break up with a couple of years before. The biggest loss of memory and concern for us was that he didn't remember breaking up with Gina and believed that they were still together.

These challenges could have been easily resolved if it were simply a matter of telling Matt the status of things and having him accept them. But his mind also struggled with "loop thinking," a condition in which his short-term memory would not retain information. Matt would ask us what time Shelly was coming home from work, then five minutes later ask the same question. He would tell us a funny joke, then tell it again within the same hour. And he would go back to believing that he was living in the past, even though we tried to correct his inaccurate memory.

In addition to his memory problems, we slowly got an inventory of the challenges he had before him that came with traumatic brain injury. Dr. Bixler had told us that we wouldn't know for sure the extent of Matt's long-term injuries until a year after the accident, and that every brain injury is different. In Matt's situation, we faced a variety of problems, some more severe than others; some less obvious to the public but not any less significant.

Matt was walking a little farther each day. By January, he had gotten to the point where he could walk pretty much anywhere, as long as he could hold on to someone's hand or arm for balance. His right arm and leg got stronger each day, but he had to continue to exercise it more than the left to help it catch up. If we took him anywhere that involved a lot of walking, we still took the wheelchair, though by the end of January, that was no longer necessary.

Part of Matt's balance problem was that he saw double, a result of the severe trauma to his head. This problem was for the most part resolved in the spring when Texas Rehabilitation Clinic finally was able to have Matt's eyes examined, and he purchased prism glasses, which corrected his double vision.

Matt's coordination and reflexes were woefully behind even mine, much less what they should have been for a young man in his twenties. We worked on this with a variety of games at home, especially his PlayStation 2 with the car-racing games. As Matt continued to race against me over the months, he gradually got better and better. Now I rarely win a race against him.

Dr. Bixler had also warned us that in a lot of ways it was as if Matt were reborn and starting over. Initially, as he began speaking, we realized that he had the maturity of a small child. We would have to explain things simply to him. The things that interested him were things that would have fascinated him as a little boy but he would have shown no interest in before the accident. In addition, in a lot of ways Matt was re-experiencing puberty. His face and back broke out in a severe case of acne, and we constantly had to treat his skin.

But in all of our re-education of Matt, the thing that made it all emotionally possible was that he had become a positive, constantly happy person. He woke up in the morning smiling and stayed that way all day. And it was obvious that he enjoyed being with us, his family.

While the daily grind of work and school drew Shelly's and my attention away from home, Missy struggled with her new volunteer job of taking care of Matt. A highly sanguine person, Matt took pride in being a young man in the fast lane, always on the go. Missy, on the other hand, was melancholy and tended to like activities she could do at home. She rarely was interested in doing something outside the home.

Before the first week was out, we realized there would be a problem.

"Matt always wants to do something, to go somewhere," she said to us one evening.

"It's boring here," he said. "There's nothing to do but sit around and watch TV."

"Well, what would you like to do?" I asked him.

Pause. "Something other than sit around here. It's boring."

I looked at him. "Like what?"

"I-don't-know," he stammered. "Something."

So we sat down with Matt and Missy and came up with a list of activities they could do together, including such things as going to the library, the zoo, walking around the mall, and taking the dogs to the park. We bought them annual passes to the zoo and a local animal preserve, and they began using them. But the conflict continued to be that Missy would rather stay home, and Matt wanted to do something active but didn't know what it was.

I had been in contact with R'Lene Mulkey since her initial interview with Matt in Harris Methodist. I found her to be not only helpful as a resource person, but encouraging as a fellow Christian. She reminded us how far Matt had come and how we needed to keep a long-term perspective. Despite both Matt's and our eagerness to get him well, she reminded us that the brain is the slowest organ in the body to heal, and recovery would take years.

R'Lene also recommended that we begin attending support groups for families of those with traumatic brain injury (TBI). The first one we attended was at Harris Methodist in February. Some of the support groups were a bit annoying, with professionals and nonprofessionals coming in with a one-size-fits-all solution to everyone's problems. But most of them were helpful in several ways. It gave us an opportunity to hear of other families, what they had been through and continued to go through, and to learn and be inspired by them. It also gave us contact with medical professionals who dealt with TBI as well as social workers and others dealing with the political aspects of getting funding.

It also gave Matt an opportunity to size himself up against those who were in similar straits. At the first meeting, Matt met a young man about his own age who had fallen off the roof of a three-story building and had head injury as well as countless broken bones. He had been injured three years before and was at about the same level of recovery as Matt. Matt met other TBI survivors in other meetings, and consistently he saw that they continued to struggle with physical and mental challenges for many years to come.

The guest speaker for the meeting at Harris Methodist was a man in his forties who had been an engineer seven years before. He had gotten kicked in the face at a karate class. The next morning he had gone to work as usual, but while sitting at his desk realized that he didn't know any of the people coming in to see him in his office. They took him to the doctor and discovered that he had sustained a brain injury from the kick. After months of treatment, he had to resign as an engineer, due to his inability to deal with the deadline pressures that came with the job. He had connected with Texas Rehabilitation Commission, who discovered that he had an aptitude for painting. He attended art school, and today he paints portraits for a living.

As we talked with others, we saw that there were people who struggled with TBI, unable to find work or continue school, and there were those who had overcome their TBI limitations and gone on to make a life for themselves. But in every case, we saw that the TBI affected their lives in one way or another for years to come, and very likely, for the rest of their lives.

R'Lene Mulkey and Texas Rehabilitation Commission paid to have a neuropsychological evaluation done with Matt in January. This day-long test was usually done one year after the accident, but R'Lene, working with Dr. Bixler, felt it would be helpful to have it as a benchmark for future evaluation to see how he had progressed.

Matt did not do well. Fatigue set in early, and he was unable to finish large sections of the test. When the evaluation came back later, it stated that he had below average intelligence and that vocational training would have modest success at best.

CHAPTER *nine*

In early February, Matt revisited Dr. Bixler in his office. This time, instead of being brought in via wheelchair, Matt walked in. The first thing Dr. Bixler noticed was how tall Matt was.

"I don't think I have ever seen you standing up," Dr. Bixler said, obviously impressed. "Once again, I have to ask you: How did a big guy like you get into that little Miata?"

Matt laughed and shook his head. "All I know is that I like them."

"Well, I am going to have to start calling you my miracle patient," Dr. Bixler continued, a gleam in his eye. He turned to me. "I got a copy of that article you wrote about Matt's accident."

I wasn't sure what he was talking about, then suddenly remembered the article in the *Record*. "How did you get a copy of that article?" I asked him.

"One of the nurses on 3-West is apparently an Adventist," he told me. "She cut it out and put it up on the bulletin board in the unit. I read it and made a copy for Matt's chart." He looked at me seriously. "I appreciated what you said there. I appreciated your perspective about how God works in ways we can't understand and that we should be willing to accept what He sends our way."

I stared at Dr. Bixler. Could this be the same physician who told us that we "shouldn't let faith get in the way of Matt's healing"?

As we struggled through our daily life, we had other people tell us how they respected us for sticking together and supporting Matt. Bob Mendenhall told me one day: "A lot of people in this community are watching you and your family. And a lot of people are inspired by what you are doing."

The love that we shared as a family didn't mean that we didn't have our moments of conflict as well. The time, energy, and financial struggle that went with taking care of Matt put a strain on Shelly's and my marriage. We seemed to have little time alone together, and when we did, the conversation almost always revolved around Matt. I was desperately trying to salvage my doctoral studies, which added to the stress. Missy and Matt continued to have conflict, and Missy, who had struggled with depression her whole life, found that her new responsibilities made it worse. One Sabbath, it all seemed to come to a head for me.

We were sitting in the first row of the back section of the Keene Adventist Church sanctuary. The elder had just called for us to kneel for prayer. I had kneeled, and Matt sat in the seat beside me.

"Dad," he whispered loudly. "I have to go to the bathroom. Now."

The whisper that was loud enough for three rows to hear, combined with the timing of it during the quietest time of the church service, set my temper off.

"Come on," I whispered back, and stood to drag Matt into the aisle and out to the lobby doors. Thankfully most of those we passed had their heads bowed in prayer and couldn't see the anger that was on my face.

Shelly, Missy, and I knew of another conflict that was in the wings. Gina had left school before the fall semester was over to go home to Iowa and spend time with her father, who was battling cancer. Before she left, while Matt was in the hospital, she introduced us to her new boyfriend. She had known Josh in academy and met him again at a reunion in Nebraska. With Matt and Gina breaking up the summer before, Gina had begun dating Josh several weeks before Matt's accident. Now we knew that Gina and Josh were planning on getting married, but Matt did not know yet.

CHAPTER *nine*

What made it hard was that Matt didn't remember the two of them breaking up, and he continued to talk to Gina as if they were still dating. We also learned that part of the unspoken reason why they had broken up was that Gina had wanted to marry Matt, and he had turned her down, stating that he wasn't ready. Since the accident, Gina reminded Matt again and again that they had broken up, but he refused to believe that it had happened.

We knew that Matt would need to know the truth soon enough, and we knew that Gina needed to be the one to tell him.

Finally, Gina phoned Matt from Iowa and told him. Matt knew that she had wanted to get married for a long time and that he had not been ready for that commitment. He wished her well and hung up.

And then Matt cried like a baby.

CHAPTER ten

Matt and Missy survived the spring semester at home together without killing each other, and soon enough it was graduation time at Southwestern Adventist University. Matt took joy in seeing his friends walk down the aisle to receive their diplomas but was sad that the friends he had gained over the past few years would be leaving the Keene area while he stayed behind. Mike was not in school but took the event as a sign that he should move back to Oregon, where his parents lived.

And Gina was graduated. She came with her parents and her fiancé, Josh, who patiently waited at a distance while Gina hugged and kissed everyone in our family at graduation. Matt grumbled the whole time that he would "tear that guy's head off" if he got the chance, but we all knew that in Matt's condition he was more likely to hurt himself than anything else.

Gina had a few items stored at our house, so we made sure Matt was over at Mike's when Gina, Josh, and her family came to pick them up. The situation was awkward, and we wished that things had worked out differently—but we were happy for Gina and Josh.

May also signaled a treat for Matt and the whole family. Suzanne Willis, who had been Matt's girlfriend for a brief time in academy and a good friend since fourth

CHAPTER *ten*

grade, was getting married in Idaho. We decided that was a good excuse for the four of us to take a vacation to Idaho as well as visit family in California. We flew into Sacramento and rented a car. Then we visited Shelly's brother Walter and his family in Lodi and my mother in Oroville before driving to McCall, Idaho, where the wedding was to take place.

It was late May, and the hot summer was rapidly approaching in Texas, but snow still covered the mountains in Idaho. After living in flat Texas for five years, we realized how much we missed the beauty of Idaho.

Matt spent some quality time with several of his academy friends. Word of his accident had gotten back to Idaho, and many of our friends were pleasantly surprised to see how well he was doing. However, it was also obvious to them that he still needed some physical therapy. And we knew that Matt's less obvious problems often took some time for a person to recognize.

Having almost lost Matt and realizing that his areas of injury weren't always evident on the surface, Shelly and I realized that we seemed overprotective of him. Matt had always been very independent, and he struggled to become that way again. On the other hand, there were many times when his body language was that of a little boy, such as holding my hand or laying his head on Shelly's shoulder. We knew that his healing would take a long time and that, more than anything else, we were glad Matt was still alive and with us. Thus we were aware of our overprotectiveness, but didn't do much to change it, at least for the time being.

Complicating the issue was the fact that Matt suffered from lack of insight, what some might call self-awareness. As time wore on, we realized that Matt did not have the ability to recognize his shortcomings. When we talked about therapy, he felt that the only thing he needed was some speech therapy. The brain injury, coupled with two months of not talking, had resulted in Matt developing a "thick tongue," which many people often equate with being mentally slow. Because of Matt's radio background, he was sensitive to this and hoped to someday go back into radio. But that was the only area with which he admitted that he needed help.

Matt was unaware of his balance problems, his lack of coordination and reflexes, the weakness on the right side of his body, and his cognitive problems, such as loop thinking and loss of short-term memory. We wanted him to have as normal and rich a life as he could possibly have yet were protective of him because of these challenges he had yet to address. His need to be independent and our need to protect him sometimes resulted in conflict.

Because Missy had spent the semester at home with Matt and because she was getting her minor in French, we agreed to let her spend six weeks taking classes at the Adventist school at Collonges, France. We felt that the time away from the pressures at home would do Missy good. Her tuition was paid through Southwestern, and she had saved up the money for airfare; so we put Missy on a flight to Geneva, Switzerland, the closest airport to her school. At first, it was difficult for her to be away. She felt both guilty leaving us at home to take care of Matt and homesick for the tightly knit family we had become. But we encouraged her to stick it out, and in less than a week she relaxed and began to enjoy herself.

I was finished with school for the summer, so Matt and I spent our days together, and Shelly joined us in the evenings. That gave me an opportunity to experience firsthand what Missy had struggled with all spring semester. If I had a day full of activities planned before Matt got up, he was content. But if I did not or had work I wanted to do around the house, Matt would mumble and grumble about "being stuck around this boring old house" and tell Shelly that evening that we had done nothing all day. We asked him a couple of times if he would like to go back to the hospital and become a patient again, but he agreed that home was preferable to that.

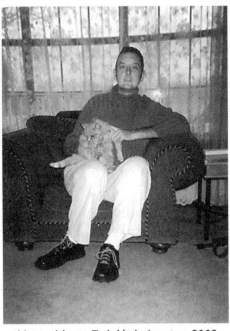

Matt with cat Twinkle in January 2003 (at home)

One of Matt's other cognitive challenges was that he no longer was able to take the initiative in starting projects. He could tell you that he wanted to do something, but couldn't tell you what it was. He was willing and able to follow instructions as long as they were very specific. But he could not find the motivation to do some of the activities that he had found joy in before the accident. For example, he had enjoyed painting as a hobby before the accident, and for months after it, he told Gina that he would paint her picture. Now, nearly two years after the accident, he is finally finishing that project.

To help him find that lost initiative and to keep a record of his physical and mental state of being during his rehabilitation, Shelly and I had bought Matt a video camera in March, using funds he was now receiving from Social Security. We justified the expenditure because he had a degree in video production. By surrounding him with equipment and facilities he was familiar with and could use in his chosen field, we reasoned, he was more likely to start using them again. This, it turn, would refresh his memory and help him prepare for joining the working world someday soon.

With his video camera, which was purchased in March, we asked him to keep a video diary. He set up the camera in his room on a tripod facing his bed, and upon our prompting, would turn it on and record the events happening to him at that time. Most of the time, he had little to talk about, because he couldn't mentally list the things that were happening and often because he wasn't really doing that much. Many of the entries in his video diary consisted of his simply saying, "I'm bored."

His boredom came to a halt when he was accepted into the outpatient rehabilitation program at Harris Methodist Hospital. Social Security benefits had finally kicked in, and with them, Medicaid benefits. Matt began visiting Harris three days a week for a half day each time. Initially, he spent time in occupational therapy, speech therapy, and physical therapy. In addition, Harris gave him an initial vocational evaluation to get a sense of what kind of job he eventually would be able to do.

Matt and I were pleasantly surprised to see that he would once again be working with many of the same people who had served as his therapists in the hospital. Jerry West was back, and she once again made sure that Matt did his very best. Those who had known Matt in 3-West were astonished at how much he had improved since he had left the hospital.

One of the devices Jerry had Matt work on was a giant metal wall-mounted plate with plastic buttons that would light up. Matt would stand facing the plate, and as the buttons would light up, he would reach up as quickly as pos-

CHAPTER *ten*

sible and hit the button before it switched off and another one lighted up. The activity could be adjusted for speed and range and could exercise his range of motion as well as his reflexes. Matt also worked on putting round and square blocks into holes to improve his dexterity. Finally, because Matt talked about wanting to go back to work at Olive Garden as a server, Jerry had Matt practice carrying a serving tray and taking orders.

The therapy that summer helped Matt improve his physical abilities and become more like his old self. More than anything, however, it was designed to see where his long-term challenges would lie and teach him compensating skills so that he could function in society as comfortably and effectively as possible.

For example, because of his short-term memory problems, Jerry pushed Matt to always carry a notepad and write everything down. This suggestion was reiterated by R'Lene Mulkey and Dr. Bixler, but Matt continued to resist, partly because he wanted to be as much like his "old self" as he could be. The argument one heard from Matt whenever this technique was suggested usually was, "Why should I? I never had to write things down before the accident."

When Mike moved to Oregon, Matt began talking about moving to Portland as well. We suspected that idea was partially because Matt had been planning to fly to Portland the day of the accident. As time went on, the idea of "moving to Portland" became more and more a perceived solution to all of Matt's problems. Despite our concerns that Matt would need to maintain a support system for years to come, he fixated on moving to Portland. Eventually we used the idea of a future move to Portland as a long-term goal for him. As long as we kept it sometime in the distant future and didn't tell him it would never happen, he was content.

Not My Son, Lord!

Little by little, Matt's maturity level improved, by now moving from childhood to that of a teen. We were reminded of his petulant nature as a thirteen-year-old and how we had often wondered how we would all survive until he became an adult.

But through it all, a new blessing appeared. Matt had fallen in love with God again. As we told him again and again of the accident, his time in TICU and 3-West, and how he lived today despite all the odds against him, Matt realized that God had spared his life. "God must have a plan for me," he said time and again.

Matt found a young-adult Sabbath School class that he really liked, and he pushed each week to be on time to Sabbath School. And even though he still fell asleep in church, the family was there together.

As the end of summer approached and we looked forward to Missy coming home from France, another problem arose.

While Matt was in the hospital, Olive Garden and other friends made donations to help us with expenses related to Matt's hospitalization and rehabilitation. Knowing that we would need all the help we could get, Shelly and I established a bank account titled the Matt Robinson Medical Fund that would be used to help us pay for things that would otherwise come out of our own pockets. In addition, in February, State Farm Insurance had written Matt a three-thousand-dollar check for his totaled Miata. Knowing that he would want to replace his car some day, we set that money aside in our own credit union account.

Funding from Social Security finally began coming to Matt in March. When they learned that Matt had received insurance money for his car, they told us that he was no longer eligible for Social Security or Medicaid, because he had additional income. Because of this policy, we had to use his car-insurance money to pay some of his medical bills.

CHAPTER ten

When summer came along, Social Security learned that we had received donations from friends in Matt's behalf. Ms. Schoenthal, our Social Security representative, told us that even though the account was in our name, any funds that benefited Matt would have to have his name on the account. Following her instructions, I took Matt to the bank and added his name to the account.

Social Security then told us to send them all statements for the account all the way back to when it was established in October. We complied. The next thing we heard from Social Security was a notice telling us that because Matt had income that had not been reported, he would have to repay all of the $3,500 that Social Security had sent him up to that point.

We did not have the money to return the Social Security payments. In addition, Shelly and I did not feel we should have to pay money back. The additional income in question consisted of donations that were made to Shelly and me to help us with our expenses. Social Security did not provide any funding until March, and Matt had bills that needed to be paid starting with his accident in October. The money only officially became Matt's income because Ms. Schoenthal insisted that he put his name on the account.

We explained the situation to Matt, but he didn't seem to understand what was going on. We knew that it would come down to a confrontation, and we hated confrontation.

I sent a letter of appeal to Ms. Schoenthal. She replied with a form letter stating that we still owed $3,500. I then sent the same letter of appeal to the main office of Social Security. I was rewarded by a letter stating that an appeal date had been set up for August 3.

On that day Shelly, Matt, and I met with the appeals judge in the offices of Social Security Administration in Cleburne.

Not My Son, Lord!

The judge led us into a small room, closed the door, and turned on a tape recorder.

"I want you to know that this is not a trial," she said, smiling. "It is simply a hearing to determine if you have grounds to appeal your case. Do you have anything you want to say to begin with?"

I was stressed, not sure what we could do against an immense bureaucracy such as the Social Security Administration. I nodded to Shelly, who sat quietly praying on the other side of the table.

"I have a letter that spells out our position," I said. "With your permission, I'd like to read it to you."

Because of the complicated nature of the situation and the numerous dates involved, I wanted to be as succinct and clear as possible. I read the letter, which explained what had happened, and asked that Social Security cancel out their claim against us while discontinuing Matt's claim to SSI and Medicaid. The judge paused.

"So you say that Ms. Schoenthal told you to put Matt's name on the account?" she asked.

"That's right," I agreed.

She paused again. "Well, in that case, I think we can go along with your proposal. In exchange for discontinuing Matt's claim to SSI and Medicaid, we will drop our claim against you."

I felt a huge weight roll off my shoulders. Not only had I worried how we would pay the debt, but I also felt like I was a criminal, cheating the government. Now I knew otherwise.

We left the Social Security office and moved on with our lives.

CHAPTER eleven

The therapists at Harris Methodist did what they could to help Matt that summer, and he made significant improvement in balance, coordination, and strength. But as the outpatient sessions came to an end, the therapists made it clear to me that many of the problems he needed to address were less obvious on the surface and yet more important.

Matt's goal was to get back to the life he had before the accident and pick up where he left off. Shelly's and my goal was a little less ambitious: to enable Matt to live an independent and happy life. We wanted him to have a job that would support him financially and to be mature and stable enough to someday marry and have a family.

The loss of Medicaid benefits did not worry me. I was grateful that they had made Matt's summer outpatient rehabilitation possible, but it seemed that continuing to meet all the conditions were more of a hassle than they were worth.

Now, at the end of August, we got a call from R'Lene Mulkey at Texas Rehabilitation Commission. "The funding has come in for Matt," she said. We set up an appointment for a few days later to talk about where we should go from there. "There is an opening at Pate Rehabilitation," she told Matt, Shelly, and me. "They would like to meet with you three and Missy to interview Matt and see if he would benefit from being in their program."

Shelly and I were thrilled that Matt would get some further rehabilitation, but Matt was less than thrilled. "I don't know what they can do for me that I can't do for myself," he said. "The only thing that's wrong with me is that my speech is a little slower than it used to be."

"Matt, how did you feel about going to outpatient rehab this summer?" I asked. "I mean, at first?"

"Well it was better than sitting at home staring at the walls," he responded.

"Did you think it would help you that much?"

"Not really."

"How do you feel now?" R'Lene asked him. "Was it worth the six weeks you were at Harris in outpatient rehab?"

Matt shrugged, then nodded. "I guess I am doing better than I was."

"Well, you need to look at this the same way," Shelly told him. "You may not see where you need to improve, but others can because they are professionals. And they will be able to help you get better."

"But I'm fine now!" he insisted.

Matt finally agreed to meet with the Pate rehab staff and discuss how it would help him. As we talked with him, we realized that his resistance had two causes. First, we already knew that part of his brain injury had affected his ability for insight, that is, he could not look at himself objectively and see that anything was wrong.

In addition, we learned that he was afraid. Afraid of leaving home and being away from his family, those who cared about him and had taken care of him twenty-four hours a day for the past several months.

We also figured out that deep down he was afraid to be around others who had more severe brain injuries than he.

CHAPTER *eleven*

The inpatient program worked with brain injury survivors at a variety of levels. Some were well on the road to recovery and were receiving vocational training to do better in the workplace. Others were severely injured and would very likely remain in Pate, or a similar facility, for the rest of their lives.

Matt was apparently afraid of being classified with those who were in the more severe category. When he was around others with brain injuries, it reminded him that he had a brain injury as well and would need to learn compensation skills for his shortcomings that he would use the rest of his life. By being around those who had not had an accident, he could try to forget that the accident ever happened.

And Shelly and I wondered if deep down he worried that we would leave him there, that he would never be able to leave Pate. We talked long and hard with Matt, and after several meetings with Pate, he agreed to join the program. What convinced him to go were two things: First, we asked him to do it for us, his parents, who had already sacrificed so much for him (a little guilt judiciously applied!), and second, Dr. Bixler told Matt that he could not get his driver's license again unless he went.

Knowing that in many ways Matt had continued to mature, but that we were still dealing with someone with the maturity of a sixteen-year-old, Dr. Bixler told us: "Don't hesitate to make me the Bad Guy. I will always be willing to give the bad news to Matt when he needs to hear it. I know how hard it is to reason with a loved one in this situation. He will thank you later."

Matt joined the Pate program in August. We took a Sunday afternoon and moved Matt up to the Pate residential house in Irving, about an hour from our house. The next day, Monday, the entire family went through orientation to the program at their offices in Dallas. Shelly was helping

Not My Son, Lord!

another hospice agency in Dallas while they looked for another director, so a couple of days a week she would finish her work in Dallas and come by Matt's house in Irving to spend time with him. I took Wednesday as my visiting days, and in the afternoon would drive up to see him. He usually arrived back in Irving about five o'clock, and I tried to time my arrival to just about the time they got there. Almost always when Shelly or I came to visit, Matt would ask us to take him to Taco Bell. With a dozen people living at the Pate house, the workers there cooked everything in bulk, and Matt often had to deal with meals of pork chops or other foods he didn't eat.

The first two weeks Matt was at Pate, he was not allowed to come home on the weekend, so it seems Matt made up for it by trying to bring his home up to him in Irving. Knowing that he would be home on weekends, and that he would be in Irving only for three months, I hesitated to take all the stuff that Matt had collected in his room, such as his computer, his TV, his PlayStation, his two turntables and mixer with table, his guitar, and his giant floor speakers. But little by little, I found myself dragging Matt's stuff up to Irving for him. I sensed that he drew comfort by having his "stuff" around him.

Fortunately, he had a very tolerant roommate. Zeb was a young man the same age as Matt, and the two of them got along terrifically. Zeb was at Pate because he suffered from epilepsy. His attacks had become so severe that physicians were forced to surgically remove part of Zeb's brain to lessen the attacks. Zeb was recovering in the Pate program and was scheduled to finish about the same time as Matt was.

As always, Matt made friends quickly. Within a week, he knew every person—both resident and staff—in the Pate house, and they knew him. When Matt joined Pate, Zeb had a seventeen-year-old girlfriend named Billy, who had been injured in an auto accident. The three of them became inseparable. Matt also grew close to a resident in her forties named Janet, who had also suffered from an auto accident. One thing that I noticed was that the younger the person was when injured, the faster his or her recovery most likely would be.

The Pate program focused primarily on preparing Matt to get into the working world. The staff had him work on a variety of problems on the computer, including math problems, word challenges, and logic questions. As his ability improved, they moved him into a different room that had distractions, such as outside noise. Eventually he was working on the computer with people and music all around him.

During the three months that Matt was at Pate, we met with his therapists at the end of each month. They talked about his progress, or lack of it, but for the most part had positive things to say about him and his ability to apply himself. For our part, whenever Matt became resistant toward the program, we reminded him that he needed to finish it successfully before Dr. Bixler would approve his driving again.

The last time we met with the therapists, we expressed concern that Matt continued to talk about moving to Portland to be with friends. We wanted him to be able to move out on his own, but we wanted there to be some sort of safety net for him, a support system until he could learn to live on his own again. More than one therapist told us that we needed to be willing to let him "fall on his face a few times" in order to learn how to live independently and what his limitations were. As parents, we knew what they were saying, but it was hard to think of him moving so far away without any support.

November marked three months that Matt had been in Pate, and he was successfully graduated from the program.

Not My Son, Lord!

The Pate program ended with Matt visiting Dr. Bixler in his office, who dutifully signed a form asking the Texas Department of Public Safety (DPS) to retest Matt on both the written and driving test for his driver's license. As I had previously agreed, I took Matt down to the DPS the day after he got back home. He talked confidently of the test, but I could tell that he was nervous. Matt passed the written test by missing only two. Then I waited while he went out with the examiner for his driving test. He returned all smiles.

"He passed," the examiner said behind him. "But I told him he needs to slow down!"

We also celebrated Matt's arrival back home by taking Zeb with the family to the amusement park Six Flags Over Texas in Irving. Missy took her friend Jessica. Determined to prove that he was back to his old self, Matt rode on the giant teacup ride—and threw up, helping him realize that his balance had not completely recovered. Zeb had a blast and was enjoying himself thoroughly until he had a seizure while we were eating at a small restaurant.

"Oh no oh no oh no oh no," he muttered, and his whole body shuddered. Shelly reached over and steadied him as he sat at the table. After a brief moment, the seizure passed, and Zeb recomposed himself.

"He had seizures so often when I was rooming with him that I don't even notice them anymore," Matt said matter-of-factly.

The six of us finished our meal and spent the rest of the evening enjoying Six Flags.

Right before Thanksgiving, I was once again privileged to invite Al Denson to give a free concert for our listeners at the end of KJCR's annual Sharathon. Zeb had heard me talk about the fact that I managed a radio station, and every time I came by or called Matt during Sharathon week, Zeb asked how the Sharathon was doing. Seeing his interest, Matt invited Zeb to go to the free concert. Both of them arrived early and answered phones as listeners called in to make pledges.

Thursday night, once again I had the responsibility of introducing the Christian performer Al Denson. I started as I always did, by bringing in my radio station staff and having them join me on the stage.

"Last year at this time, I told you about a young man who was involved in a near-fatal auto accident. He has had a very difficult and long road since then, and he has a long way still to go. But I am thrilled to tell you that he is here with us tonight. Matt Robinson, can I have you stand please?"

Matt stood in the front section of the Keene sanctuary, and the room thundered with applause. I stood in the front, overwhelmed with a flood of memories from the past year, and overwhelmed with gratitude for a loving God who had carried us through the ordeal my family had survived—and continued to survive. I stood for a long moment, allowing the applause to wash over me, and then slowly joined them in clapping my hands.

After the concert, I brought Matt up to meet Al Denson.

"Al, this is—," I never got to finish the sentence. Al Denson grabbed Matt's hand and shook it.

"It is pleasure to meet you," he said. "You are looking great, considering all you have been through." He smiled broadly. "Isn't God good?"

Matt nodded. "He sure is."

And I stood behind the two of them in silent, sober agreement.

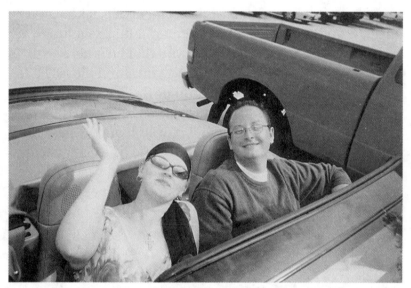

Matt today in his new Miata with his cousin, Meghan

Epilogue

The difficult part in writing a story such as ours is that, while the beginning is relatively obvious, the ending is not. Recovering from brain injury, like sanctification, is the work of a lifetime. Unfortunately, not all who fight the good fight following traumatic brain injury are overcomers. Instead, the battle is in stretching the boundaries of one's short-term limitations to the maximum, learning what one's long-term challenges are, and developing skills and mechanisms that will help one live in the world as effortlessly and inconspicuously as possible.

For all that most victims of traumatic brain injury want is to do what the rest of us take for granted: go to school, work at a fulfilling, reasonably well-paying job, find a spouse, rear kids, and live as full and complete a life as possible. And speaking from experience, sometimes when you are close to losing a life or an ability, it makes you appreciate it that much more.

Throughout this unexpected adventure that started with Matt's accident, my family and I have looked at this as a physical and financial ordeal, but more than anything, a spiritual journey. I have had a tendency in the past to take things for granted, most specifically, the joy of being with my wife and children and the many, many ways that God has blessed me and continues to bless me every day of my

Not My Son, Lord!

life. The accident forced Shelly and me to shorten the focus of our lives. Those days in the TICU waiting room led us to move from planning weeks and months ahead to a universe measured in a single day. For I have learned that God gives us one day at a time, and we should be grateful for the day we have, because there are no guarantees that tomorrow will ever arrive.

I also feel I have a little better understanding of the phrase Ellen White uses when she speaks of a "primitive godliness." Living on the edge makes one lean on God harder than ever before and forces one to realize that the harder we lean on Him, the better off we will be. God has strong shoulders. Often our biggest problem is that we aren't willing to use that strength.

As we close in on the two-year mark since Matt's accident, he has progressed much further than any of the medical professionals involved with his case could have predicted. Most strangers, upon first meeting Matt, are unaware that he was involved in a serious accident. However, when he is tired, such as when he has been working all day, his speech begins to get slurred again, his movements get slower, and his thinking processes slow down.

In January 2004, Matt returned to work as a server at Olive Garden. He worked there for several months until it was determined that he just couldn't maintain the work speed he had before the accident. At this writing, he is working part time as an Olive Garden host, showing diners to their tables. He doesn't make as much money as he once did, but he still works among his friends.

In November 2003, Matt had gotten his driver's license again, and with our help, took out a loan for a used automobile to replace his totaled Miata. After lots of shopping and negotiation with his parents, Matt purchased

Epilogue

another Miata, this time a black one. Many people, when hearing what car he drives now, are amazed that Matt would go back to the same type of vehicle that he drove in the accident. But upon further scrutiny of the accident and how it had occurred, I have decided that most likely the auto itself was not the reason Matt hit his head. The airbag deployed properly, the seatbelt was used, but Matt had a tendency to put his shoulder harness under his arm, saying that having it over his shoulder "bothered him." Because the shoulder harness was improperly used, it didn't prevent his head from smashing into the top of the windshield. Since he started driving again, Matt has faithfully worn his shoulder harness the way it was designed to be worn.

Matt recently realized one of his dreams; he has been accepted into a Master in Fine Arts program in film at the Miami International University of Art and Design for April 2005. Matt continues to struggle with verbal skills and the ability to choose words he needs to express himself. He also has trouble reading. But the school he has been accepted to is part of the same Art Institute system Matt attended in Seattle, and they tend to be less book-oriented and more hands-on in their approach. We have learned not to underestimate Matt's ability to do something once he puts his mind to it. With lots of help from the school's disability tutoring center, and the grace of God, we will have to see how Matt does. At this point, we know that anything is possible, especially when it involves Matt.

The accident has led Matt to a fresh face-to-face relationship with his Creator. He has found a young-adult Sabbath School he enjoys, and is faithful in attending church, even though he is likely to fall asleep during the sermon, as he had since the accident. He knows that he is more than lucky;

in his own words, "I know that God has something special for me to do. Otherwise why would He have saved me like that?"

With each additional day that comes between us and October 17, 2002, the date of the accident, Matt becomes more and more his old self. He struggles with many of the same challenges that those in his age group struggle with. He is looking for a girlfriend. He is looking for a better job. He wonders if he will do OK when he goes back to school. He wants to have fun. He wants to be taken seriously.

Matt officially said Goodbye to Dr. Bixler in April 2004, when Dr. Bixler told him that he had progressed beyond his official need for therapy. Dr. Bixler, the person who had told Shelly and me to "not let our faith get in the way of Matt's healing," told Matt this: "I have been calling you my 'miracle patient.' But I can't take credit for your progress. It's not really a miracle, because you have a lot of people on your side, especially a God who loves you very much."

R'Lene Mulkey said Goodbye with the following comment: "Matt, you will continue to have people telling you what your limitations are. But we know better. Support from a loving Christian family and your own sheer determination has taken you this far—and will take you places that will surprise even you. I see you going on to graduate school and excelling."

Before the accident happened, Shelly and I were beginning to talk about the reality of having our kids leave home and were slowly embracing the concept of the "empty nest." As Christian parents, we had realized that our children had grown beyond the point of having us tell them what to do, and we saw that there comes a time when all Christian parents can do for their children is pray for them.

Epilogue

It is a helpless feeling, but in a lot of ways it is a healthy thing to do. Having Matt on death's door in the hospital reinforced that need to pray for him. Now, as Matt talks about moving to Florida, we are once again confronted by that limitation.

And the reality is, all Christian parents come to the same point when they have to let go and let God. We have a tendency to want to do it ourselves; God is asking us to trust Him with our children. Because, after all, they're really just on loan to us by Him.

Shelly and I are just grateful that God gave us a second chance.